# CHAIR YOGA FOR WEIGHT LOSS

*A Collection of 60+ Low-Impact Exercises for Seniors and Beginners to Lose Weight While Sitting on a Chair*

# TABLE OF CONTENTS

# Thanks
*for Your Purchase!*

As a token of appreciation, I'm excited to share some exclusive resources to enhance your yoga journey and make it even more rewarding.

## What's Included:

- **30 Days Challenge Yoga Video Course: a s**pecially designed video course to guide you through a 30-day chair yoga challenge. These sessions will help you build consistency, improve flexibility, and experience the transformative benefits of yoga at your own pace.

- **Printable Chair Yoga Journal:** this journal is the perfect companion to your yoga practice. Use it to track your progress, set goals, and reflect on your daily sessions. It's a simple yet powerful tool to stay motivated and mindful throughout your journey.

## How to Access Your Gift?

To download your gifts, simply **scan the QR code provided on Page 103 of this book**. The QR code will take you to a dedicated page where you can access both the video course and the printable journal.

Thank you for embarking on this chair yoga journey with me. I hope these gifts inspire you to take your practice to the next level and enjoy the many benefits of yoga!

# Chapter 1: Introduction to Chair Yoga

## Understanding Chair Yoga

Chair yoga is an accessible form of yoga that has been tailored specifically for individuals who find traditional yoga poses challenging or for those who prefer a gentler approach to their exercise routine. It incorporates the use of a chair as a support tool, enabling participants to perform a variety of yoga poses and stretches while seated or using the chair for balance and stability. This method of yoga is particularly beneficial for seniors or beginners who are concerned about the strain and flexibility demands of conventional yoga practices.

The essence of chair yoga lies in its adaptability and inclusiveness. Exercises can be modified to accommodate the physical limitations or health concerns of the practitioner, making it an ideal choice for individuals with mobility issues, chronic pain, or those recovering from injuries. The chair provides a stable base, reducing the risk of falls and allowing for increased confidence during practice.

**Chair yoga exercises** focus on improving flexibility, strength, balance, and posture while also encouraging better breathing habits. The routines often include a variety of movements that target the upper body, lower body, and core, ensuring a comprehensive workout that can aid in weight management and overall physical health. Additionally, chair yoga emphasizes mindfulness and relaxation techniques, which can lead to reduced stress and improved mental well-being.

For those looking to incorporate chair yoga into their weight loss journey, it's important to understand that while chair yoga can be a gentle form of exercise, it can still effectively contribute to calorie burn and muscle toning. The key is consistency and gradually increasing the duration or intensity of the practice as one becomes more comfortable and stronger. Integrating chair yoga into a daily routine can not only aid in achieving physical fitness goals but also enhance the quality of life by promoting a sense of harmony between the mind and body.

Safety is paramount in chair yoga, as with any exercise program. It is advisable to choose a sturdy, non-slip chair and to wear comfortable clothing that allows for unrestricted movement. As beginners, especially seniors, embark on this journey, it might also be beneficial to practice under the guidance of a certified chair yoga instructor who can provide personalized adjustments and ensure that the exercises are performed correctly.

In summary, chair yoga offers a versatile and safe option for individuals seeking a low-impact exercise routine. Its benefits extend beyond physical health, touching on emotional and mental well-being, making it a holistic approach to fitness that is accessible to a wide range of individuals, including seniors and beginners. By incorporating chair yoga into their lifestyle, practitioners can enjoy the numerous health benefits of yoga without the need for extensive physical strength or flexibility, making it a valuable tool for weight loss and improved overall health.

## Benefits of Chair Yoga for Seniors

Chair yoga presents a multitude of benefits specifically tailored to meet the needs of seniors, making it an invaluable practice for those seeking a gentle yet effective form of exercise. **Flexibility** is one of the first notable benefits; as we age, our joints and muscles can become stiff and less pliable. Chair yoga helps to counteract this stiffness, promoting a greater range of motion and reducing the risk of injury. This is crucial for maintaining daily activities and independence. **Strength** is another key benefit. The exercises in chair yoga are designed to build muscle strength gently and safely, focusing on core, arms, and legs, which are essential for balance, posture, and overall mobility.

**Balance** improvements are a significant advantage of regular chair yoga practice. Falls are a common concern among the elderly, leading to injuries and a decrease in quality of life. By strengthening the muscles and improving flexibility, seniors can enjoy better stability and a reduced risk of falls. **Mental health** benefits should not be overlooked. Chair yoga incorporates breathing and meditation techniques that can help reduce stress, anxiety, and depression, promoting a sense of well-being and relaxation. This aspect of chair yoga is especially beneficial for seniors who may be dealing with the psychological impacts of aging or isolation.

**Social interaction** is another important benefit. Joining chair yoga classes offers a sense of community and provides an opportunity for socialization, which is vital for emotional health and can combat feelings of loneliness. **Accessibility** is a key factor that makes chair yoga so appealing to seniors. It can be practiced anywhere, from the comfort of one's home to community centers, requiring minimal equipment and space. This makes it an ideal exercise option for those with mobility issues or limited access to traditional yoga studios.

**Pain management** is a crucial benefit for many seniors. Chair yoga can help alleviate chronic pain conditions such as arthritis, back pain, and fibromyalgia by gently stretching and strengthening the body. This can lead to a reduced need for medications and can improve overall quality of life. **Heart health** is also positively affected by regular chair yoga practice. The combination of physical exercise and stress-reduction techniques can help lower blood pressure, reduce cholesterol levels, and improve overall cardiovascular health.

In summary, chair yoga offers a comprehensive approach to fitness that addresses many of the physical and mental health challenges faced by seniors. Its low-impact nature, combined with the potential for social interaction and mental health benefits, makes it an ideal form of exercise for the elderly population, helping them to maintain and even improve their quality of life.

## How Chair Yoga Promotes Weight Loss

Chair yoga promotes weight loss through a series of low-impact exercises that stimulate the metabolism, enhance muscle tone, and improve cardiovascular health without putting undue stress on the body. For seniors and beginners, especially those concerned about the physical demands of conventional exercise routines, chair yoga offers a practical and effective solution to weight management. The exercises are designed to increase the heart rate gently, facilitating calorie burn in a manner that respects the body's limitations and needs. This is particularly important for individuals with joint issues or those recovering from injury, as the seated nature of these exercises minimizes the risk of strain or further injury.

**Muscle toning** is an essential component of weight loss, and chair yoga addresses this through targeted movements that engage the core, arms, legs, and back. Building muscle mass is crucial as it increases the resting metabolic rate, meaning the body burns more calories even when at rest. The various poses and stretches incorporated into chair yoga sequences are specifically chosen to activate and strengthen these muscle groups in a balanced and harmonious way.

**Flexibility and mobility** improvements, though often overlooked, play a significant role in weight loss. Enhanced flexibility can lead to better posture and movement efficiency, which in turn can make it easier and more comfortable to engage in a variety of physical activities. By reducing stiffness and increasing range of motion, chair yoga helps to break down barriers to exercise, encouraging more frequent and prolonged physical activity.

**Breathwork** in chair yoga also contributes to weight loss. The deep, mindful breathing techniques taught in chair yoga sessions improve oxygenation of the body, boost energy levels, and enhance metabolic processes. This increased oxygen intake supports the body's natural detoxification processes, aiding in digestion and helping to regulate appetite. The calming effect of breathwork can also reduce stress-induced cortisol levels, which are known to contribute to weight gain, particularly in the abdominal area.

**Consistency and accessibility** are key factors in the effectiveness of chair yoga for weight loss. Because chair yoga can be practiced virtually anywhere and requires minimal equipment, it is easier for individuals to incorporate into their daily routine. Regular practice is essential for sustained weight loss, and the convenience of chair yoga supports the development of a consistent exercise habit. The adaptability of chair yoga exercises means that as individuals become stronger and more flexible, they can gradually increase the intensity of their workouts, leading to continued improvement in fitness and further weight management benefits.

The combination of these elements—muscle toning, improved flexibility and mobility, effective breathwork, and the ability to maintain a consistent practice—makes chair yoga an excellent option for those seeking to lose weight, particularly seniors and beginners. By engaging in chair yoga, individuals can enjoy the dual benefits of enhancing their physical health while also embarking on a journey of mindful movement that supports mental and emotional well-being.

# Chapter 2: Preparing for Chair Yoga

## Setting Realistic Goals

Embarking on a chair yoga regimen for weight loss requires **setting realistic goals** that are achievable and tailored to your individual needs and capabilities. It's crucial to acknowledge that weight loss and improving fitness levels are gradual processes, especially when incorporating a gentle form of exercise like chair yoga. To establish a foundation for success, begin by evaluating your current physical condition and any limitations you might have. This self-assessment will guide you in defining clear, attainable objectives.

**Short-term goals** are an excellent starting point. These could include completing a full chair yoga session without taking extra breaks, mastering a specific pose, or practicing chair yoga a certain number of times per week. These immediate objectives serve as stepping stones, building your confidence and motivation as you achieve them.

**Long-term goals** require a broader perspective. Consider what you wish to achieve in the next six months to a year. This might involve losing a specific amount of weight, noticeably improving your flexibility and balance, or integrating chair yoga into your daily routine for sustained health benefits. Remember, these goals should be challenging yet realistic, pushing you to progress while still considering your physical limitations and lifestyle.

Incorporating **SMART criteria**—Specific, Measurable, Achievable, Relevant, and Time-bound—into your goal-setting process can significantly enhance your chances of success. For instance, a SMART goal could be, "I will attend chair yoga classes three times a week for the next three months to improve my balance and flexibility." This goal is specific (attending chair yoga classes), measurable (three times a week), achievable (considering current fitness levels and time availability), relevant (improves balance and flexibility, contributing to overall weight loss and health), and time-bound (set for the next three months).

**Tracking progress** is another essential aspect of achieving your goals. Keep a journal or use a digital app to record your chair yoga sessions, including any improvements in poses, reductions in stress levels, or weight loss achievements. This record not only keeps you accountable but also allows you to visibly see your progress, providing encouragement and motivation to continue.

**Adjusting goals** as needed is part of the process. You might find that some objectives are too ambitious or too easy, or perhaps your physical or personal circumstances change. Regularly review and adjust your goals to ensure they remain aligned with your capabilities and aspirations.

Remember, the primary aim of incorporating chair yoga into your life is to enhance your overall well-being. While weight loss may be a significant motivator, the benefits of chair yoga extend to improving mental health, increasing flexibility, and building strength. Celebrate all achievements, no matter how small, and view each as a step toward a healthier, more balanced life.

## Creating a Comfortable Space

Creating a comfortable space for your chair yoga practice is essential to ensure that you can focus on your exercises without distractions and with the utmost safety. First, select a chair that is sturdy and stable, without wheels, to prevent any movement that could lead to injuries. The chair should have a firm seat that allows your feet to rest flat on the floor when seated, and your knees should form a 90-degree angle. This positioning helps maintain proper posture and balance during your practice.

The area around your chair should be clear of any obstacles or sharp objects to create a safe radius for movement. You'll need enough space to extend your arms and legs freely in all directions. Ideally, this space should be quiet, well-ventilated, and have a pleasant temperature, making your practice more enjoyable and helping you to stay focused.

Lighting plays a significant role in creating a calming atmosphere. Natural light is preferable, but if that's not possible, choose soft, warm lighting that illuminates your space without causing glare or harsh shadows. This type of lighting can help enhance your mood and concentration levels.

Consider the surface you'll be practicing on. A non-slip floor or a yoga mat placed under your chair can provide additional stability, especially for poses that require more balance or when your feet are off the ground. If you're on a carpet, ensure the chair is stable and won't sink into the pile when you're seated.

Personalize your space with elements that promote a sense of calm and happiness. This could be a small indoor plant, a piece of artwork, or anything that brings you joy and enhances your sense of well-being. The goal is to make this space inviting and something you look forward to using daily.

Sound can also impact your practice. If you find silence distracting, consider playing soft, instrumental music or nature sounds to help you relax and focus. Alternatively, if you're easily distracted by noise, earplugs or noise-canceling headphones can be useful tools to maintain your concentration.

Temperature control is another aspect to consider. Being too hot or too cold can distract from your practice. Aim for a comfortable temperature that allows you to relax and move freely. Lightweight, breathable clothing can help regulate your body temperature and ensure comfort throughout your session.

Finally, keep any necessary accessories, such as water, a towel, or any props you might use like blocks or straps, within easy reach. This allows you to stay hydrated and comfortable without having to interrupt your practice to retrieve items.

By taking the time to create a comfortable and personalized space for your chair yoga practice, you're investing in your health and well-being. This dedicated space can become a sanctuary for physical and mental rejuvenation, enhancing the benefits of your chair yoga routine and making it an enjoyable part of your daily life.

# Necessary Equipment and Safety Tips

For those embarking on the chair yoga journey, having the right equipment is essential to ensure both safety and effectiveness of your practice. Here's a comprehensive list of necessary equipment along with safety tips to keep in mind:

1. **Sturdy Chair**: Choose a chair without wheels, with a straight back, and no arms. This ensures stability and allows for a range of movements without restriction.

2. **Yoga Mat**: Place a yoga mat under your chair to prevent it from sliding on the floor during your exercises, enhancing your safety.

3. **Comfortable Clothing**: Wear loose, comfortable clothing that doesn't restrict your movement. Avoid belts, heavy fabrics, or anything that can hinder your yoga practice.

4. **Water Bottle**: Stay hydrated throughout your practice. Keep a water bottle nearby to sip water as needed, especially important for seniors to prevent dehydration.

5. **Yoga Blocks and Straps**: These can help modify exercises to your level of flexibility and comfort. Blocks can be used to support your hands or feet, while straps can help in extending your reach and maintaining poses.

6. **Non-slip Socks**: To prevent your feet from slipping, especially when performing standing poses or movements that require foot stability.

**Safety Tips**:

- **Check the Chair**: Before each session, ensure the chair is stable and sturdy. If it wobbles or feels unstable, replace it.

- **Listen to Your Body**: Never push yourself into pain or discomfort. Chair yoga is meant to be gentle and accessible. If a pose feels too challenging, ease up or try a modified version.

- **Keep Space Clear**: Ensure the area around your chair is clear of any obstacles that you might bump into or trip over during your practice.

- **Focus on Your Breath**: Breathing is a core part of yoga. Pay attention to your breath as you move through the exercises. It should be steady and controlled, not strained or rushed.

- **Warm-Up**: Begin each session with a warm-up to prepare your body. This can include simple seated stretches or breathing exercises.

- **Consult with a Professional**: If you have any pre-existing health conditions or concerns, consult with a healthcare provider or a certified yoga instructor specialized in chair yoga before starting. They can offer guidance and modifications specific to your needs.

By adhering to these equipment recommendations and safety tips, you can create a supportive and safe environment for your chair yoga practice, allowing you to focus on your health, flexibility, and weight loss goals.

# Chapter 3: The Power of Breathing

## Breathe Your Way to Better Health

Breathing, often overlooked, is a fundamental aspect of chair yoga and a powerful tool for enhancing health and facilitating weight loss. Proper breathing techniques can significantly improve oxygenation in the body, boost metabolism, and reduce stress levels, all of which are crucial for seniors and beginners aiming to lose weight through low-impact exercises. The essence of breathing in chair yoga is not just about the inhalation and exhalation of air but about how these processes are harnessed to improve physical and mental well-being.

**Deep Diaphragmatic Breathing**, a cornerstone of yoga breathing practices, involves breathing deeply into the lungs, allowing the diaphragm to move downwards, causing the abdomen to expand. This technique enhances lung capacity, stimulates lymphatic flow to aid in detoxification, and activates the parasympathetic nervous system, promoting relaxation and stress reduction. Practicing this form of breathing can lead to more efficient oxygen exchange and increased energy levels, both vital for an effective weight loss journey.

**Box Breathing**, also known as square breathing, involves inhaling, holding the breath, exhaling, and holding again, each for an equal count of four. This method is particularly beneficial for calming the mind, reducing anxiety, and improving concentration. For seniors, this can be a powerful technique for managing stress, which is often a barrier to weight loss.

**Alternate Nostril Breathing** is another technique that involves alternating the flow of air through the nostrils by gently closing one nostril while breathing through the other. This practice balances the left and right hemispheres of the brain, calms the nervous system, and can improve sleep patterns, thereby supporting weight loss efforts by reducing stress and enhancing overall well-being.

**4-7-8 Breathing** is a technique that emphasizes the length of the exhale compared to the inhale, promoting relaxation and stress relief. By inhaling for a count of four, holding the breath for seven counts, and exhaling for eight counts, this technique helps in calming the mind and reducing cravings, which can be particularly beneficial for weight management.

**Lion's Breath** involves a forceful exhalation, which can help in releasing tension and stress, improving vocal and respiratory strength, and stimulating the metabolism. This practice, characterized by a distinctive exhalation sound, can be both energizing and therapeutic, offering a unique way to enhance the chair yoga experience.

Incorporating these breathing exercises into a regular chair yoga routine can significantly impact one's health and weight loss journey. It is recommended to start with a few minutes of these breathing practices at the beginning or end of a chair yoga session, gradually increasing the duration as comfort with the techniques grows. Remember, the goal is not to perform these exercises to perfection but to find a rhythm and pace that feels comfortable and beneficial for your body and mind. Engaging in these practices regularly can lead to profound changes in both physical and mental health, supporting weight loss and contributing to a greater sense of well-being.

# Essential Breathing Exercises for Mind and Body

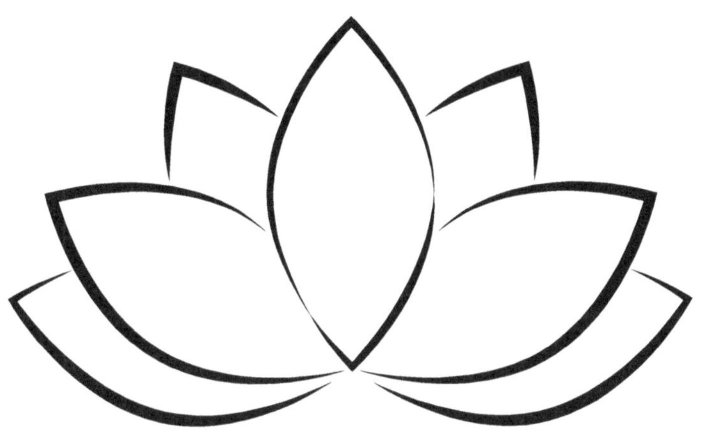

Scan the QR code to view the 5 exercises included in this section.

# Deep Diaphragmatic Breathing

**PURPOSE:** To enhance lung capacity and promote relaxation by engaging the diaphragm in deep breathing. This exercise aids in stress reduction and improves oxygen flow throughout the body, which can support weight loss efforts by improving metabolic rate and energy levels.

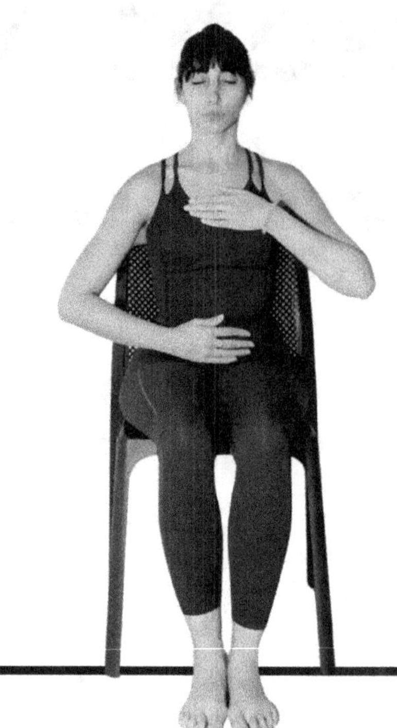

## PREPARATION

- Sit comfortably on a chair with your back straight and feet flat on the floor.
- Place one hand on your chest and the other on your abdomen. This will help you feel the movement of your diaphragm during the exercise.
- Relax your shoulders and try to clear your mind, focusing solely on your breathing.

## EXECUTION

1. Slowly inhale through your nose, feeling your abdomen expand with your hand rising, while your chest remains relatively still.
2. Pause for a moment when you feel your abdomen is fully expanded.
3. Exhale slowly through your mouth, pursing your lips slightly, and use the hand on your abdomen to gently press and help expel air.
4. Focus on making your exhale twice as long as your inhale to fully engage the diaphragm and encourage relaxation.
5. Repeat this breathing pattern for 3 to 5 minutes, gradually increasing the duration as you become more comfortable with the exercise.

### Tips and Advice to Avoid Common Mistakes

Ensure you are breathing through your diaphragm, not shallowly from your chest. The hand on your abdomen should move more than the hand on your chest.

# Box Breathing

**PURPOSE:** To calm the mind, reduce stress, and improve concentration by regulating the breath. This technique can be particularly beneficial for seniors looking to manage stress levels and enhance focus.

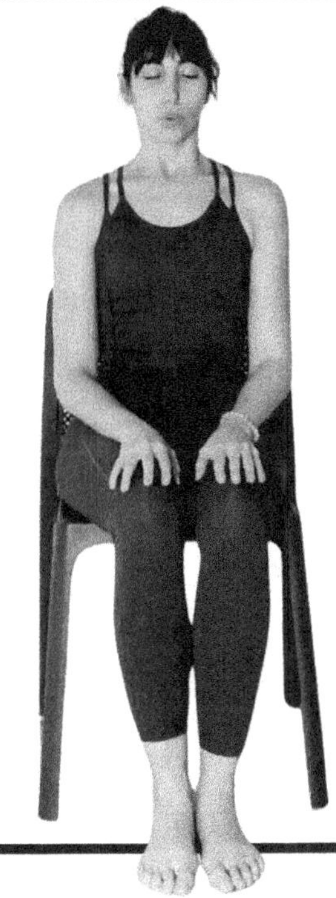

## PREPARATION

- Choose a comfortable, stable chair with a straight back.
- Sit up tall, feet flat on the floor, hands resting gently on your lap. Close your eyes to minimize distractions and focus more on your breathing.
- Close your eyes to minimize distractions and focus more on your breathing.

## EXECUTION

1. Inhale slowly and deeply through your nose to a slow count of four, feeling your chest and belly rise as you fill your lungs with air.
2. Hold your breath for a count of four. Try to avoid clenching your muscles; keep your body relaxed.
3. Exhale slowly through your mouth for a count of four, consciously releasing all the air from your lungs and belly.
4. Hold your breath out for a count of four before inhaling again.
Repeat this cycle for several minutes, aiming for a total of 5-10 cycles.

**Tips and Advice to Avoid Common Mistakes**

If you find holding your breath for four counts too challenging, start with shorter counts and gradually increase as you become more comfortable.

# Alternate Nostril Breathing

**PURPOSE:** To enhance respiratory function, balance the nervous system, and reduce stress and anxiety by alternately breathing through each nostril. This exercise is particularly beneficial for improving focus and calming the mind, making it ideal for weight loss efforts by reducing stress-induced eating.

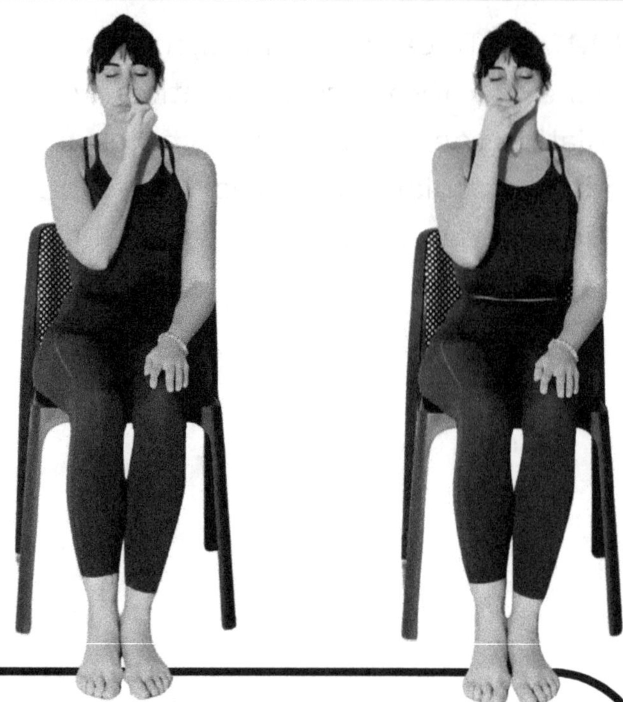

## PREPARATION

- Sit comfortably in your chair with your back straight and feet flat on the floor.
- Relax your left palm comfortably on your lap and your right hand just in front of your face.
- Using your right hand, make a "peace sign" with your middle and index finger, folding them towards your palm, leaving your thumb, ring, and pinky fingers extended.

## EXECUTION

1. Gently close your right nostril with your right thumb.
2. Inhale slowly and deeply through your left nostril.
3. Close your left nostril with your ring and pinky fingers, releasing your thumb from your right nostril.
4. Exhale slowly through your right nostril.
5. Inhale through your right nostril.
6. Close the right nostril with your thumb, releasing the ring and pinky fingers from your left nostril.
7. Exhale through your left nostril.

This completes one cycle.
Aim for 5-10 cycles, focusing on smooth and deep breaths.

**Tips and Advice to Avoid Common Mistakes**

Ensure you are seated in a stable chair without wheels to maintain balance during the exercise.

# 4-7-8 Breathing

**PURPOSE:** To calm the mind, reduce anxiety, and improve oxygen delivery to the brain and body, promoting relaxation and aiding in weight management by reducing stress-induced eating.

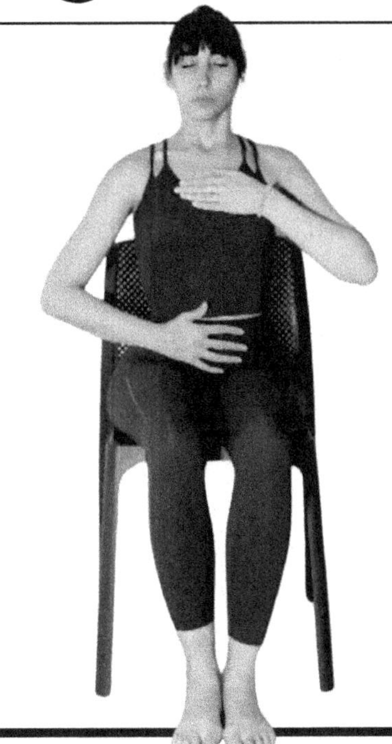

## PREPARATION

- Sit comfortably in your chair with your back straight and feet flat on the floor.
- Place one hand on your belly and the other on your chest to feel the movement of your breath.
- Close your eyes gently to minimize external distractions.

## EXECUTION

1. Exhale Completely: Begin by letting all the air out of your lungs through your mouth, making a whoosh sound.
2. Inhale Through the Nose: Close your mouth and inhale quietly through your nose to a mental count of four.
3. Hold Your Breath: Hold your breath for a count of seven.
4. Exhale Through the Mouth: Exhale completely through your mouth, making a whoosh sound to a count of eight.
5. Repeat: This completes one cycle. Repeat the cycle three more times for a total of four breaths.

## Tips and Advice to Avoid Common Mistakes

Concentrate on your breathing. If your mind wanders, gently bring your attention back to the counts of 4-7-8.

# Lion's Breath

**PURPOSE:** To release tension in the face and neck, improve respiratory function, and energize the mind and body. This exercise is particularly beneficial for seniors looking to manage stress and enhance their lung capacity in a gentle yet effective way.

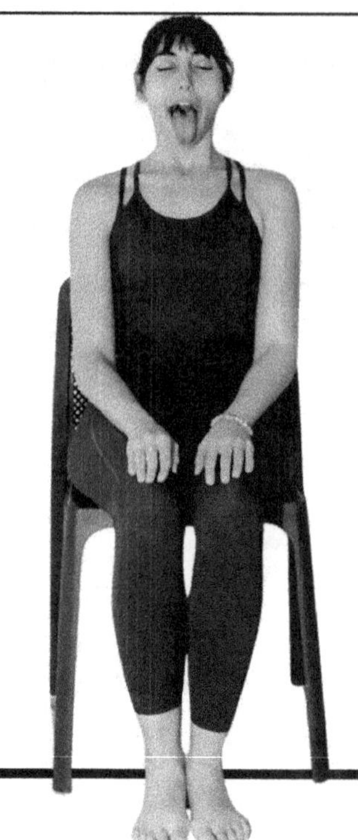

## PREPARATION

- Sit comfortably in your chair with your spine straight and feet flat on the floor.
- Place your hands on your knees or in your lap, whichever feels more natural.
- Relax your shoulders away from your ears and gently close your eyes to focus on your breath.

## EXECUTION

1. Inhale deeply through your nose, filling your lungs completely.
2. Open your mouth wide, stick out your tongue as far as you can towards your chin.
3. Exhale forcefully through your mouth, making a "ha" sound from deep within your throat.
4. As you exhale, envision releasing all the tension and negativity from your body.
5. Close your mouth and breathe in gently through your nose to return to your starting position.
6. Repeat this process for 3 to 5 breaths, gradually increasing the number of repetitions as you become more comfortable with the exercise.

### Tips and Advice to Avoid Common Mistakes

If sticking out your tongue feels uncomfortable, you can modify the exercise by keeping the tongue behind your teeth.

# Chapter 4: Chair Yoga for Weight Loss and Toning

Embarking on a journey with chair yoga for weight loss and toning involves integrating various exercises that target key areas of the body to promote fat loss and muscle strength. The beauty of chair yoga lies in its adaptability, making it a perfect fit for seniors and beginners who are cautious about engaging in more strenuous forms of exercise. By focusing on low-impact, seated movements, individuals can effectively work towards their weight loss goals without the risk of injury or strain on the joints.

Starting with **Warm-Up and Simple Movements**, it's crucial to prepare the body for the session ahead. A series of gentle stretches and mobility exercises, such as the Seated Mountain Pose and Seated Cat-Cow Stretch, help to loosen up the muscles and increase blood flow. These initial movements are designed not only to warm up the body but also to introduce participants to the practice of mindful movement and breathing, which are core components of yoga.

**Basic Core Engagement and Balance** exercises are next, focusing on strengthening the core muscles from a seated position. The core is the foundation of all movement, and a strong core contributes to better posture, reduced back pain, and improved balance. Exercises like the Seated Core Twist and Chair Plank are essential for building core strength. They are performed slowly and with control, emphasizing the importance of breath in synchrony with movement.

Transitioning into exercises for **Upper Body Strength and Flexibility**, the focus shifts to the arms, shoulders, chest, and upper back. Strengthening these areas can significantly improve daily functional movements, such as lifting and reaching. The Seated Shoulder Rolls and Seated Arm Raises are examples of movements that enhance upper body mobility and strength, which are vital for maintaining independence in daily activities.

For **Lower Body Strength and Mobility**, incorporating exercises like Seated Ankle Circles and Seated Calf Raises addresses the lower extremities. Strengthening the legs and improving ankle mobility are crucial for balance and walking, which are essential for a senior's independence and overall health.

Each of these exercises is performed with the aid of a sturdy chair to ensure safety and stability. The chair not only provides support but also allows for modifications of traditional yoga poses to accommodate various levels of flexibility and mobility. This adaptability makes chair yoga an inclusive practice, ensuring that everyone, regardless of their physical condition, can participate and benefit from the exercises.

Incorporating these exercises into a regular routine can lead to significant improvements in physical health, contributing to weight loss and enhanced muscle tone. The key is consistency and gradually increasing the intensity of the exercises as strength and confidence grow. By focusing on controlled movements and breathwork, participants can maximize the benefits of their chair yoga practice, improving not only their physical health but also their mental well-being.

To further amplify the benefits of chair yoga, incorporating **Full-Body Movements for Fat Burning and Mobility** is essential. These exercises are designed to increase the heart rate gently, promoting cardiovascular health and aiding in fat loss. Movements such as the Seated Full-Body Stretch and Seated Arm and Leg Reach not only engage multiple muscle groups simultaneously but also enhance coordination and mobility. By engaging in these dynamic exercises, participants can enjoy a comprehensive workout that stimulates fat burning while minimizing the risk of injury.

The **Relaxation and Recovery** segment of the practice is equally important. After engaging in the active part of the session, dedicating time to wind down and stretch is crucial for muscle recovery and stress reduction. Exercises like the Seated Relaxation Pose and Seated Gentle Twist aid in releasing tension from the body and calming the mind. Incorporating mindful breathing during this phase further enhances relaxation, promoting a sense of well-being and mental clarity.

Safety is paramount in chair yoga, especially for seniors and beginners. It is advised to maintain a slow and steady pace, focusing on proper form and alignment to prevent strain or injury. Utilizing props such as yoga blocks and straps can aid in achieving poses safely, making the practice more accessible. Participants are encouraged to listen to their bodies, modifying poses as needed to accommodate their comfort levels.

Regular participation in chair yoga sessions can lead to significant health benefits, including improved strength, flexibility, balance, and mental health. Moreover, the weight loss and toning effects of these exercises can contribute to a healthier lifestyle, promoting longevity and enhancing quality of life.

To maximize the benefits of chair yoga, consistency is key. Starting with shorter sessions and gradually increasing the duration and intensity allows the body to adapt without overwhelming it. Encouraging a routine practice can help build the habit, making it easier to incorporate chair yoga into daily life. With time, participants may notice improvements not only in their physical health but also in their emotional and mental well-being, underscoring the holistic benefits of this gentle yet effective form of exercise.

By integrating these exercises into a regular chair yoga routine, individuals can enjoy a safe, effective, and comprehensive approach to weight loss and toning. The adaptability of chair yoga makes it an ideal choice for those seeking a low-impact form of exercise that accommodates their physical limitations while offering tangible results.

# Warm-Up and Simple Chair Yoga Movements

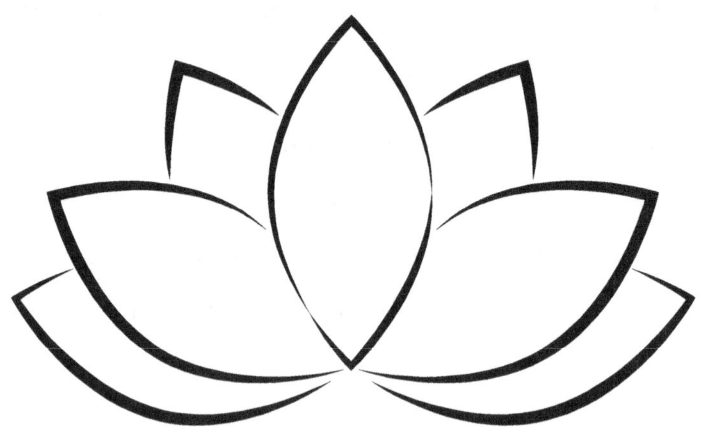

Scan the QR code to view the 8 exercises included in this section.

# Seated Mountain Pose

**PURPOSE:** To improve posture, increase spine flexibility, and promote a sense of grounding and stability. This foundational pose serves as a great starting point for chair yoga practice, helping to align the body and prepare the mind for further exercises.

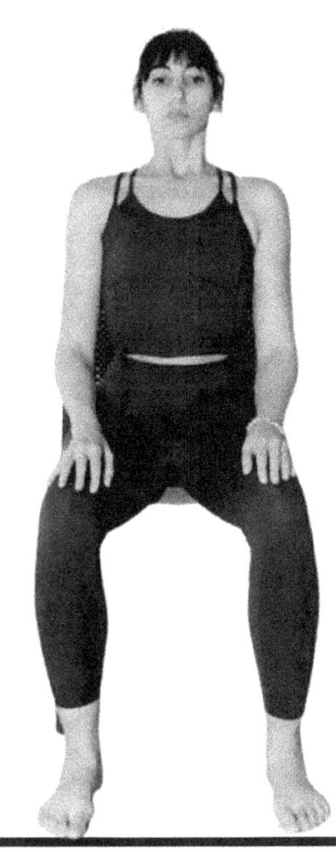

## PREPARATION

- Choose a sturdy chair without arms, and sit at the front edge. Ensure your feet are flat on the floor, hip-width apart.
- Rest your hands on your thighs or knees, palms down.
- Straighten your spine as if a string is pulling you up from the top of your head, but keep your shoulders relaxed.

## EXECUTION

1. Inhale deeply, elongating your spine further, feeling each vertebra stretch upward.
2. As you exhale, gently press your sit bones into the seat of the chair, grounding yourself.
3. Keep your chin parallel to the floor, and gaze directly forward with a soft focus.
4. Engage your abdominal muscles slightly to support your spine.
5. Hold this pose for 5 to 10 deep breaths, focusing on maintaining a tall, straight posture and steady breathing.
6. With each inhale, imagine growing taller. With each exhale, feel more grounded and stable.

### Tips and Advice to Avoid Common Mistakes

Ensure your feet are firmly planted on the ground. If your feet don't comfortably reach the floor, place a book or block under them for support.

# Seated Cat-Cow Stretch

**PURPOSE:** To improve spinal flexibility and stimulate the abdominal organs, enhancing digestion and promoting relaxation.

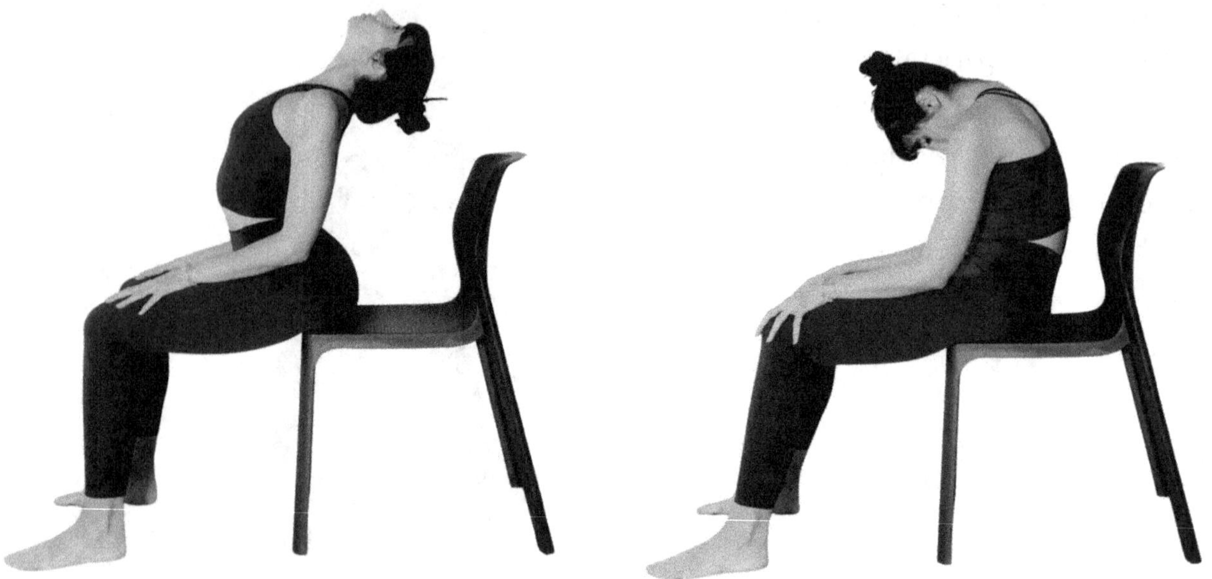

## PREPARATION

- Choose a sturdy chair without arms, and sit at the edge with your feet flat on the ground, hip-width apart.
- Place your hands on your knees or thighs, keeping your spine straight and shoulders relaxed.
- Take a few deep breaths to center yourself and prepare for the exercise.

## EXECUTION

1. Inhale: Slowly arch your back, pushing your stomach forward, tilting your pelvis back, and looking up towards the ceiling. This is the "Cow" position.
2. Exhale: Gently round your spine, tucking your chin to your chest, pulling your belly button towards your spine, and curving your back towards the chair. This is the "Cat" position.
3. Flow: Smoothly transition between the Cow and Cat positions, moving with each breath. Inhale as you arch your back and exhale as you round it.
4. Repeat: Continue this flowing movement for 3-5 minutes, focusing on the sensation in your spine and the rhythm of your breath.

### Tips and Advice to Avoid Common Mistakes

Engage Your Core: Ensure you are engaging your abdominal muscles throughout the exercise to support your spine.

# Seated Forward Bend

**PURPOSE:** To gently stretch the spine, shoulders, and hamstrings, promoting flexibility and relieving tension in the back.

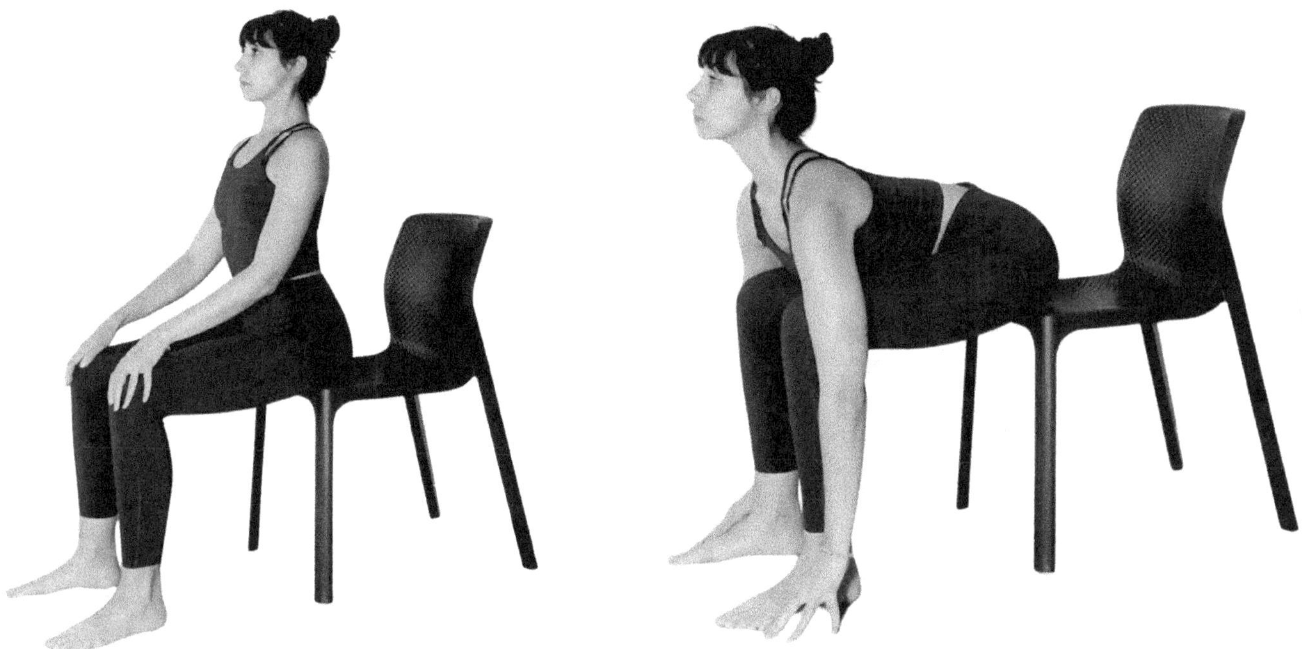

## PREPARATION

- Choose a stable chair without arms and sit at the edge with your feet flat on the ground, hip-width apart.
- Keep your back straight, shoulders relaxed, and hands resting on your thighs.
- Take a few deep breaths to center yourself before beginning the exercise.
·

## EXECUTION

1. Inhale deeply and lengthen your spine, imagining a string pulling you up from the crown of your head.
2. As you exhale, slowly hinge forward from your hips, keeping your back straight.
3. Slide your hands down your legs towards your feet, going only as far as comfortable without rounding your back.
4. Hold the position for a few deep breaths, feeling a gentle stretch in your back and legs.
5. To come out of the pose, inhale and slowly lift your torso back up to sitting position, using your hands on your thighs for support if needed.
6. Repeat the movement 2-3 times, gradually deepening the stretch with each repetition.

# Seated Spinal Twist

**PURPOSE:** To increase flexibility and strength in the spine, improve digestion, and promote better posture.

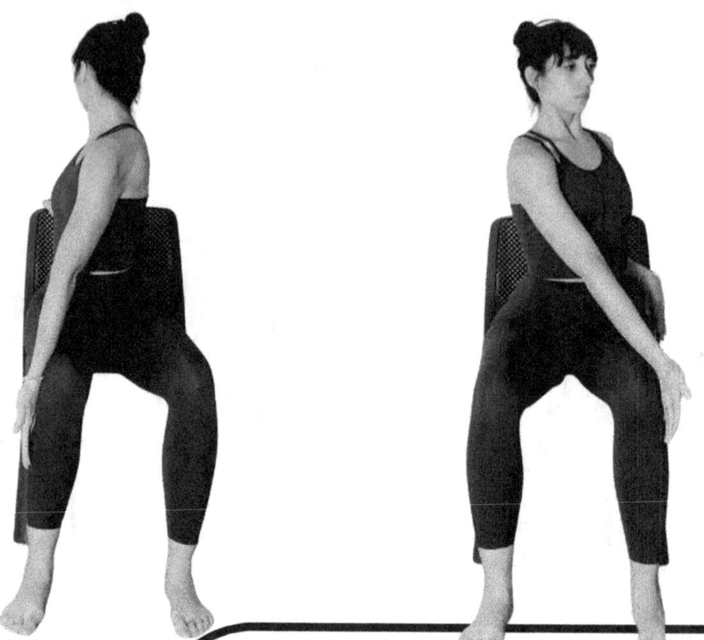

## PREPARATION

- Choose a sturdy chair without arms and sit towards the front edge so that both feet are flat on the ground, hip-width apart.
- Sit up tall, extending your spine, and engage your core muscles slightly to maintain a straight posture.
- Rest your hands on your thighs or knees.

·

## EXECUTION

1. Inhale deeply and, as you exhale, gently twist to the right from the bottom of your spine. Think of wringing out your waist like a wet towel.
2. Place your left hand on the outside of your right knee and your right hand wherever it feels comfortable, perhaps on the seat of the chair or behind you for support.
3. Keep your hips facing forward and allow the twist to originate from the midsection of your body.
4. Hold this position for 3-5 deep breaths, focusing on lengthening your spine with each inhale and deepening the twist with each exhale.
5. Inhale to return to center, then repeat the twist on the left side.

### Tips and Advice to Avoid Common Mistakes

Beginners should perform this exercise slowly and increase the depth of the twist gradually over time.

# Seated Side Bend

**PURPOSE:** To stretch and strengthen the muscles along the sides of your torso, improving flexibility and aiding in the reduction of waistline fat.

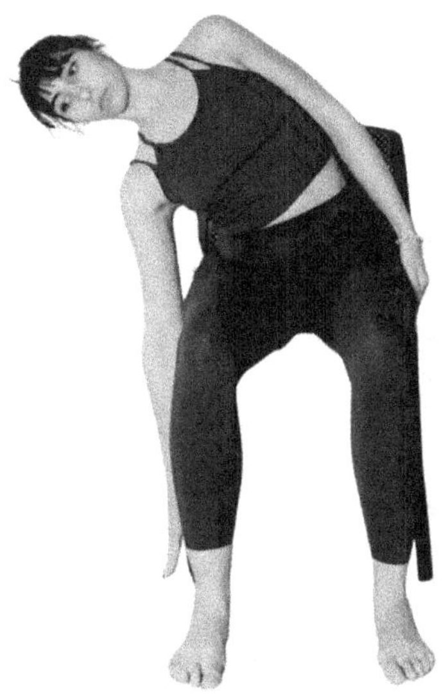
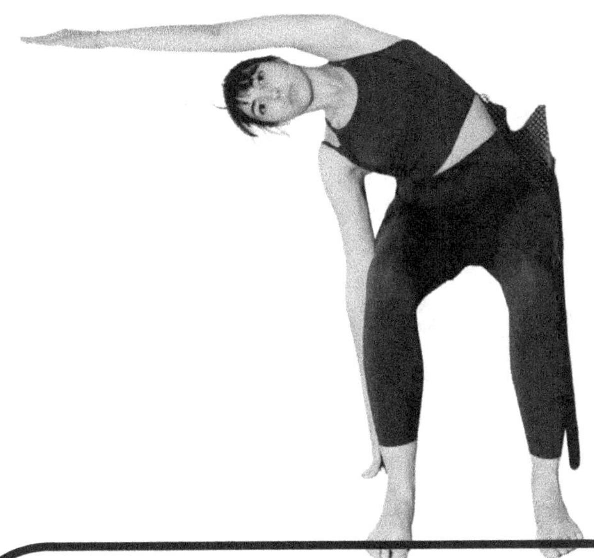

## PREPARATION

- Sit upright in a sturdy chair without arms, feet flat on the ground, and knees aligned over your ankles.
- Place your hands on the sides of the chair seat for stability.
- Engage your core muscles gently to support your spine.

## EXECUTION

1. Inhale deeply and exhale as you lean your torso to the right, sliding your right hand down the chair.
2. Keep your left hip grounded and extend your left arm overhead in a straight line.
3. Hold for 3-5 breaths, elongating on inhales and deepening the stretch on exhales.
4. Inhale to return upright, then repeat on the left side.
5. Alternate sides for 3-5 repetitions, maintaining smooth, controlled breathing.

**Tips and Advice to Avoid Common Mistakes**

Avoid jerky movements or using momentum to lift your leg. The movement should be controlled and deliberate to maximize muscle engagement and reduce the risk of injury.

# Seated Leg Lifts

**PURPOSE:** To strengthen the quadriceps and improve stability in the knees and hips, aiding in weight management by increasing muscle tone and metabolism.

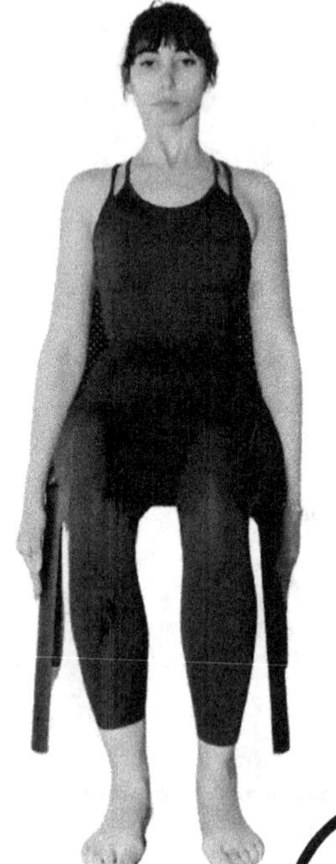
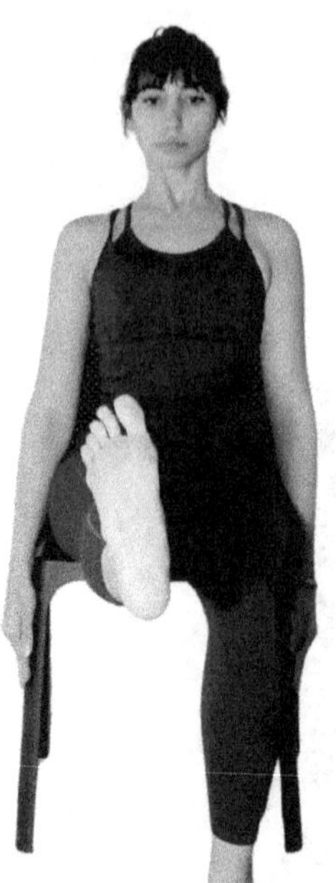

## PREPARATION

- Choose a sturdy chair without arms and sit at the edge with your back straight and feet flat on the ground, hip-width apart.
- Place your hands on the sides of the chair for balance.
- Engage your core muscles to maintain good posture throughout the exercise.

## EXECUTION

1. Slowly extend one leg out in front of you as straight as possible, keeping the other foot flat on the ground.
2. Flex your foot so that your toes are pointing back towards you.
3. Hold the leg lift for a count of 3-5 seconds, feeling the engagement in your thigh.
4. Slowly lower your leg back to the starting position with control.
5. Repeat the movement with the other leg.
6. Aim for 10-15 repetitions on each leg, gradually increasing the number as you gain strength.

### Tips and Advice to Avoid Common Mistakes

Keep your back straight and avoid leaning backward as you lift your leg. This ensures the focus remains on the leg muscles and helps prevent strain on your back.

# Seated Arm Circles

**PURPOSE:** To improve shoulder mobility and flexibility, promote upper body circulation, and gently engage the core muscles, contributing to overall posture improvement and aiding in the weight loss process by activating multiple muscle groups.

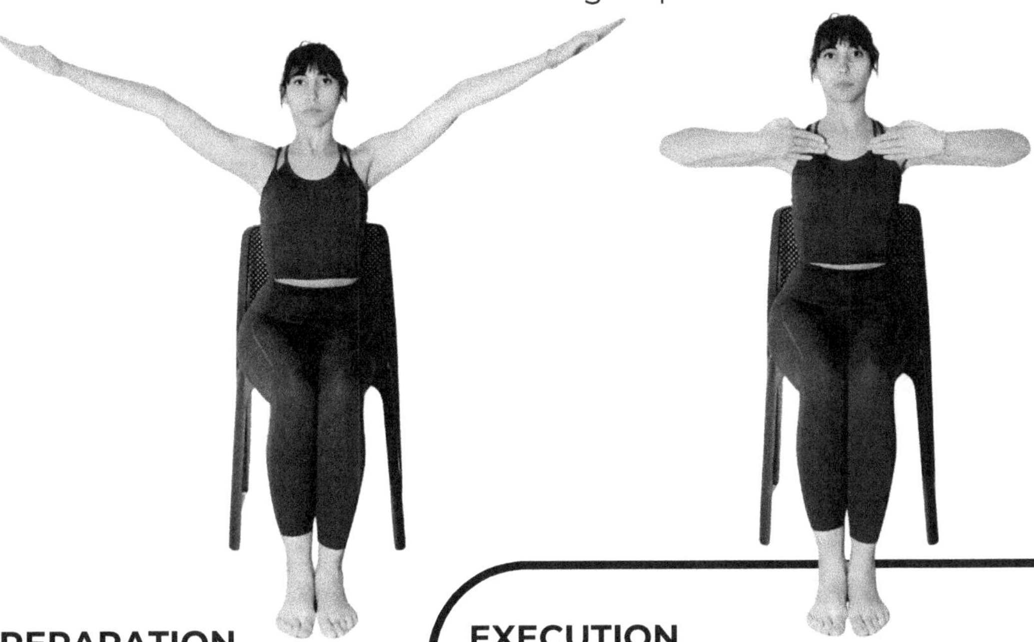

## PREPARATION

- Choose a sturdy, armless chair and sit with your feet flat on the ground, hip-width apart.
- Keep your back straight, engaging your abdominal muscles slightly to support your spine.
- Extend your arms to the sides at shoulder height, palms facing down.

## EXECUTION

1. Begin by slowly circling your arms forward in small circles, gradually increasing the size of the circles as you become more comfortable.
2. Continue this motion for 30 seconds, focusing on keeping the movement smooth and controlled.
3. Pause and reverse the direction of your circles, starting small and increasing in size, continuing for another 30 seconds.
4. Ensure your movements are initiated from the shoulders, not just the wrists or elbows.
5. Keep your neck relaxed and your gaze forward, avoiding any strain in the neck or shoulders.

### Tips and Advice to Avoid Common Mistakes

Avoid shrugging your shoulders towards your ears; keep the shoulder blades drawn down and back throughout the exercise.

# Seated Marching

**PURPOSE:** To improve circulation, strengthen leg muscles, and enhance cardiovascular health, all while seated comfortably.

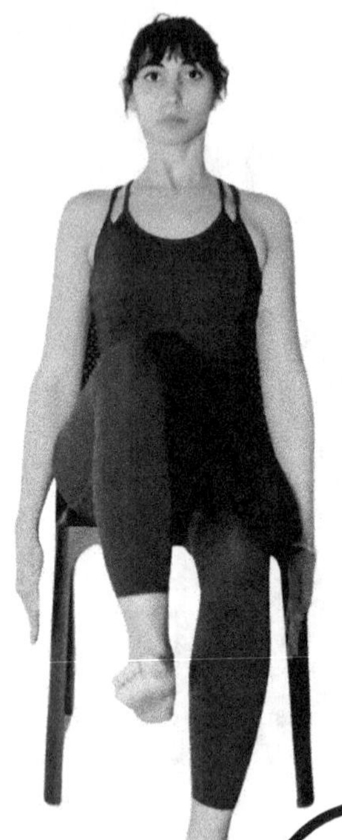

## PREPARATION

- - Choose a sturdy chair without wheels, preferably one with a straight back to support your posture.
- Sit at the edge of the chair with your back straight, feet flat on the floor, and hands resting on your thighs or the sides of the chair for balance.

## EXECUTION

1. Engage your core and sit tall, ensuring your back isn't touching the backrest.
2. Lift your right knee towards your chest as high as comfortably possible, keeping your foot flexed.
3. Lower your right foot back to the floor and immediately lift your left knee towards your chest.
4. Continue alternating legs at a steady pace, simulating a marching motion while seated.
5. Aim for 1-2 minutes of continuous seated marching, gradually increasing the duration as your endurance improves.

### Tips and Advice to Avoid Common Mistakes

To increase the challenge as you progress, consider adding ankle weights or increasing the speed of your marches, ensuring you maintain proper form.

# Core Engagement and Balance Exercises

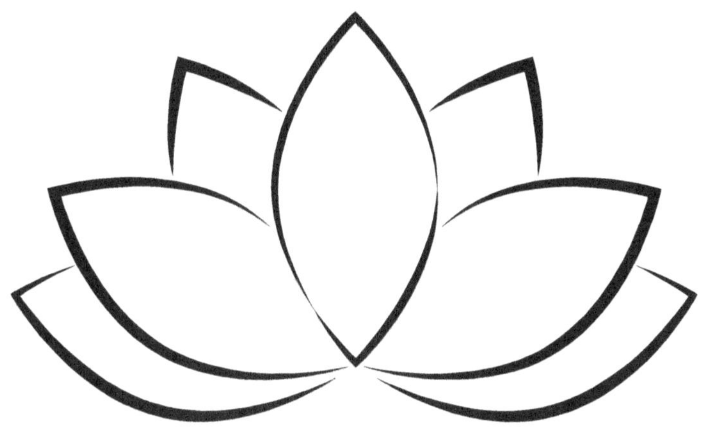

**Scan the QR code to view the 10 exercises included in this section.**

# Twist and Stretch

**PURPOSE:** To improve hip flexibility, deepen spinal twists, and enhance balance and posture while releasing tension in the lower back.

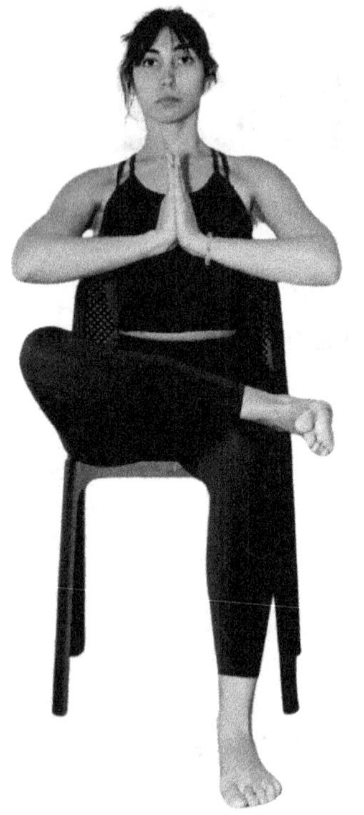 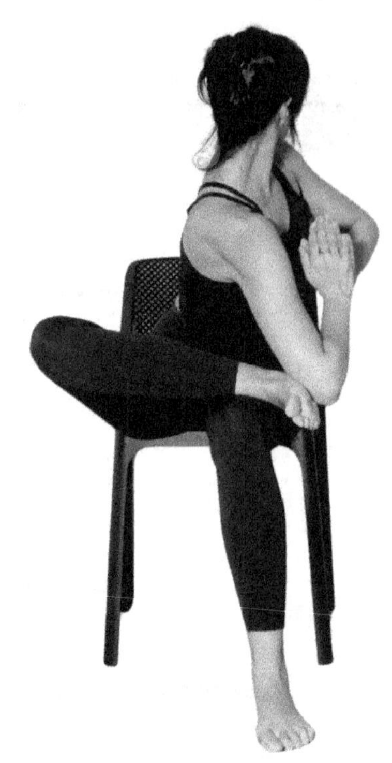

## PREPARATION

- Sit comfortably on a sturdy chair with your back straight and feet flat on the floor.
- Ensure enough space for a cross-legged position.

## EXECUTION

1. Sit tall with your feet flat on the floor and hands resting gently on your thighs. Take a deep breath to center yourself.

2. Cross your right ankle over your left thigh, forming a figure "4" with your legs. Press your palms together in front of your chest in a prayer position. Maintain an upright posture and breathe deeply.

3. Rotate your upper body to the right, placing your left elbow gently against your right knee. Keep your hands in a prayer position. Feel the twist through your spine and hold for a few breaths.

4. Unwind your twist and bring your right foot back to the floor. Repeat the sequence on the opposite side

# Chair Plank

**PURPOSE:** To strengthen the core muscles, improve posture, and enhance balance without standing.

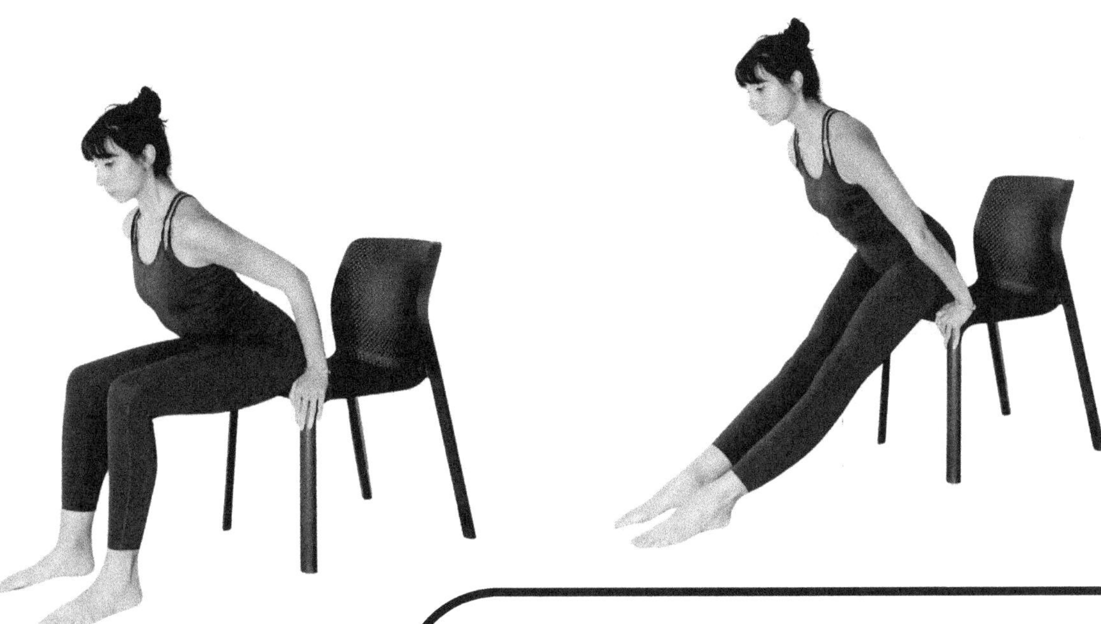

## PREPARATION

- Sit on the edge of a sturdy, armless chair with your feet planted firmly on the ground, hip-width apart.
- Place your hands on either side of the chair seat, gripping the edges for support.
- Lean slightly forward from your hips, keeping your back straight and your core engaged.

## EXECUTION

1. Press down into the chair with your hands, engaging your arms, shoulders, and core muscles.
2. Lift your buttocks slightly off the chair, keeping your feet flat on the floor.
3. Extend your legs forward, so your body forms a straight line from your head to your heels, similar to a plank position on the floor.
4. Hold this position for 10-20 seconds, maintaining a tight core and steady breathing.
5. Carefully lower your buttocks back to the chair and relax.
6. Aim for 2-3 repetitions, gradually increasing the hold time as your strength improves.

**Tips and Advice to Avoid Common Mistakes**

Avoid sagging your hips; keep your body in a straight line to fully engage the core muscles.

# Seated Bicycle Crunches

**PURPOSE:** To engage and strengthen the core muscles, including the abdominals and obliques, in a safe, seated position.

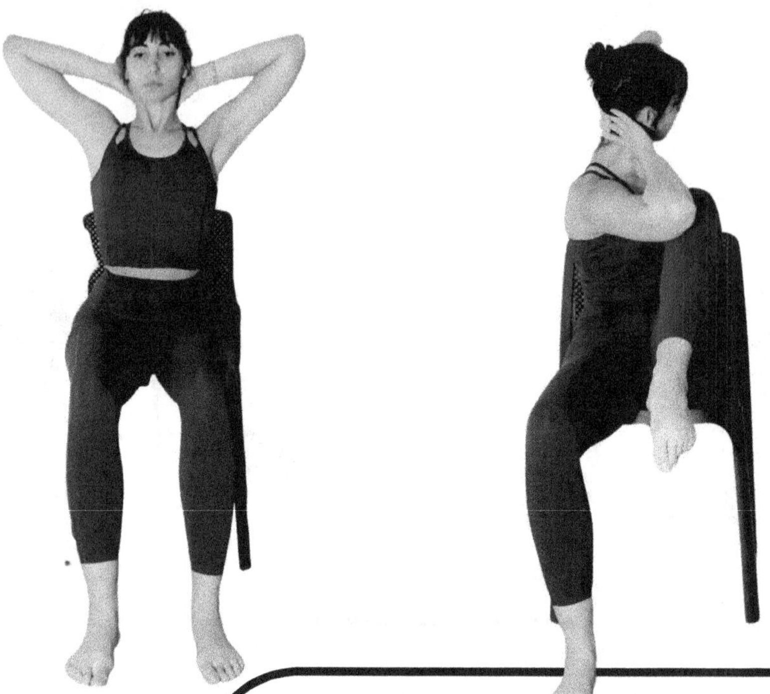

## PREPARATION

- Sit on a sturdy, armless chair, feet flat on the floor.
- Place hands behind your head with elbows wide, or cross them over your chest for comfort.
- Lean back slightly with a straight spine to engage your core.

## EXECUTION

1. Lift your right knee towards your chest.
2. At the same time, twist your torso so your left elbow moves towards the lifted knee, engaging your oblique muscles.
3. Return to the starting position and repeat the movement with your left knee and right elbow, completing one rep.
4. Aim for 10-15 reps on each side, focusing on slow, controlled movements to maximize core engagement.
5. Keep alternating sides for 2-3 sets, resting briefly between sets.

### Tips and Advice to Avoid Common Mistakes

Start with fewer repetitions and sets, gradually increasing as your strength and endurance improve.

# Seated Figure Four Stretch

**PURPOSE:** To open the hips, improve flexibility, and release tension in the lower back and glutes.

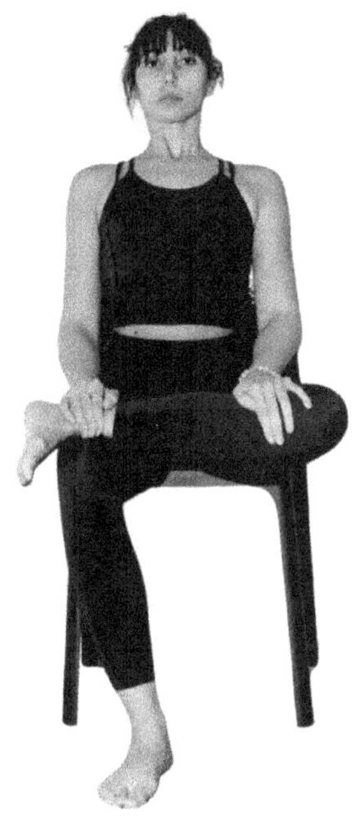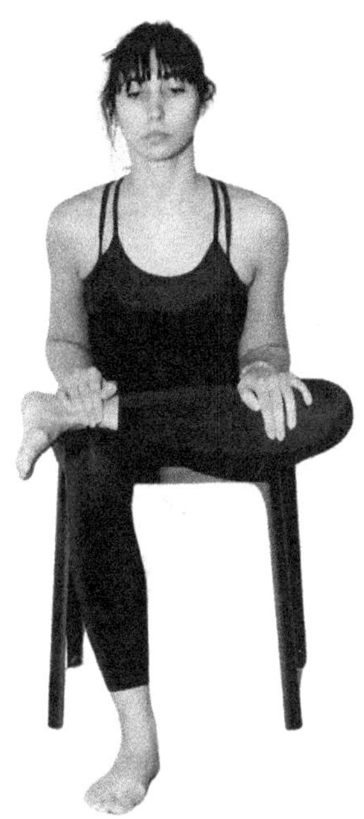

## PREPARATION

- Sit comfortably on the edge of a sturdy chair with your feet flat on the floor and your back straight.
- Place your hands on your thighs to help maintain stability.
- Take a few deep breaths to relax and center yourself before starting.

## EXECUTION

1. Sit upright on the chair with your back straight, feet flat on the floor, and arms relaxed at your sides. Breathe deeply to center yourself.
2. Cross your right ankle over your left thigh, forming a figure "4" with your legs. Keep your back straight and your hands resting on your right knee and ankle for support. Hold for a few breaths.
3. Lean your torso forward slightly, maintaining a straight back, to deepen the stretch in your right hip and glute. Breathe deeply and hold the position for a few seconds.
4. Return to the starting position and repeat the same steps on the opposite side.

# Seated Knee Tucks

**PURPOSE:** To engage and strengthen the core muscles, including the abdominals and lower back, while promoting balance and stability from a seated position.

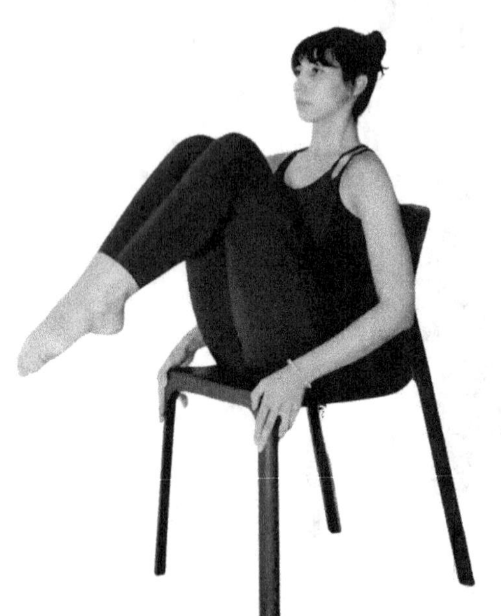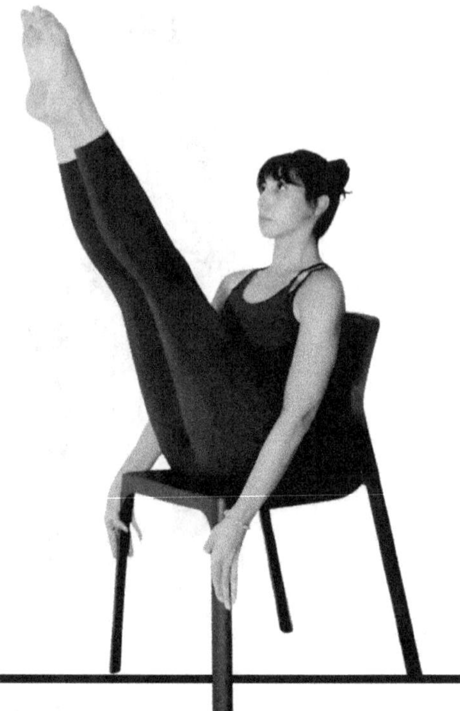

## PREPARATION

- Select a chair without arms that offers stability and allows your feet to rest flat on the ground with knees bent at a 90-degree angle.
- Sit towards the front of the chair so that you have enough space to lean back without touching the backrest.
- Place your hands on the sides of the chair for support, gripping firmly.

## EXECUTION

1. Engage your core muscles by drawing your navel towards your spine.
2. Lean back slightly, keeping your back straight and maintaining a slight angle from your hips to your shoulders.
3. Lift both feet off the ground, bringing your knees towards your chest.
4. Extend your legs out in front of you, keeping them elevated, then pull your knees back towards your chest.
5. Perform 8-10 repetitions of extending and tucking your knees, focusing on maintaining a strong, engaged core throughout the movement.
6. After completing your set, carefully place your feet back on the ground and return to an upright seated position.

# Seated Russian Twists

**PURPOSE:** To engage and strengthen the core muscles, including the abdominals and obliques, while seated.

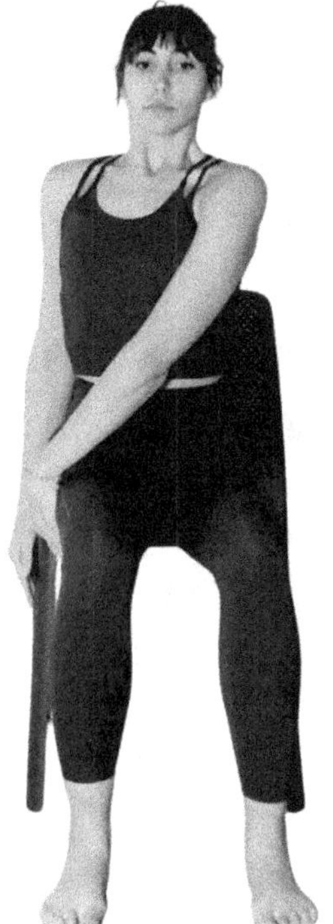 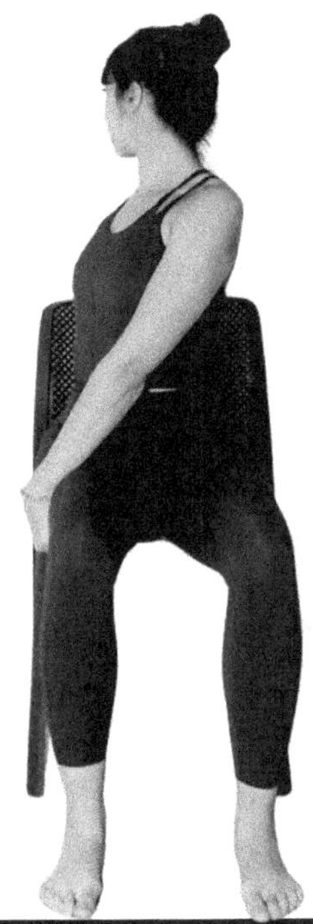

## PREPARATION

- Sit on the edge of a sturdy, armless chair with your feet flat on the ground, hip-width apart.
- Keep your back straight and engage your core muscles.
- Place your hands behind your head with your elbows wide, or cross your arms over your chest, whichever feels more comfortable.

## EXECUTION

1. Exhale and gently twist your torso to the right, aiming to bring your left elbow towards your right knee. Keep your hips and legs facing forward; the movement should come from your core.
2. Inhale as you slowly return to the center, maintaining an upright posture.
3. Exhale and repeat the twist to the left side, bringing your right elbow towards your left knee.
4. Continue alternating sides for 10-15 repetitions on each side, focusing on controlled, deliberate movements.
5. Keep your movements smooth and avoid rushing; the emphasis is on core engagement and balance rather than speed.

# Seated Side Leg Lifts

**PURPOSE:** To strengthen the muscles on the sides of the hips and thighs, improve balance, and enhance core stability, which is crucial for maintaining mobility and supporting weight loss efforts through increased muscle engagement.

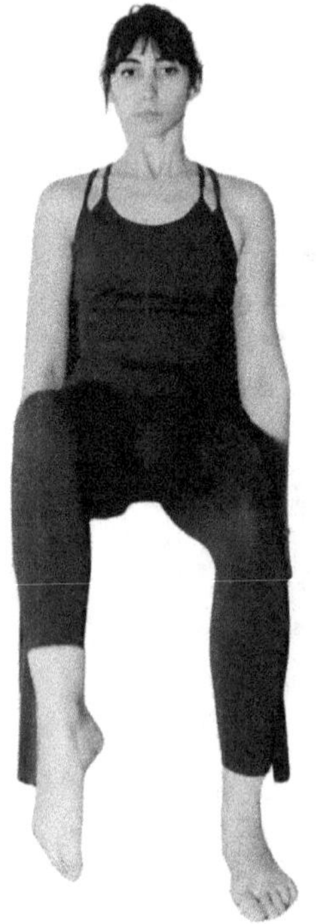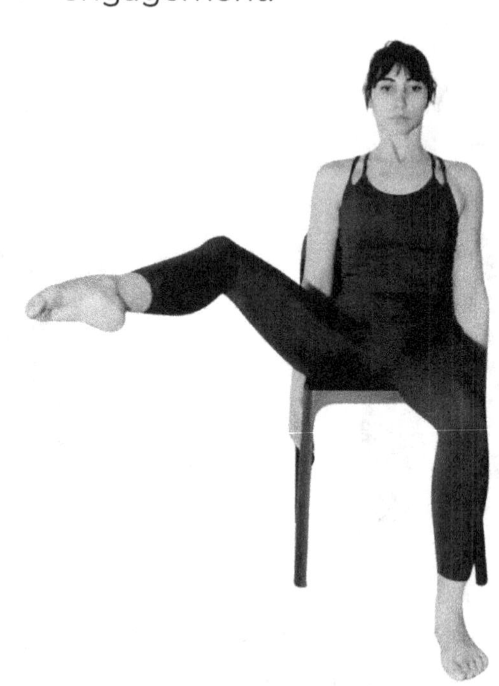

## PREPARATION

- Sit in a sturdy, armless chair with your back straight and feet flat on the floor, spaced hip-width apart.
- Engage your core by gently pulling your belly button towards your spine to provide support for your lower back.
- Place your hands on the sides of the chair seat or on your thighs for balance.

## EXECUTION

1. Shift your weight slightly to your right side, keeping your right foot firmly on the ground.
2. Slowly lift your left leg to the side, keeping the leg straight but not locked at the knee.
3. Lift the leg as high as comfortably possible without tilting your torso to the side; aim for a height where you can maintain balance and form.
4. Hold the lift for 2-3 seconds, then slowly lower your leg back to the starting position.
5. Perform 10-15 repetitions on the left side before switching to lift your right leg in the same manner.
6. Aim to complete 2-3 sets on each side, depending on your comfort and ability.

# Seated Heel Raises

**PURPOSE:** To strengthen the calf muscles, improve ankle stability, and promote circulation in the lower legs, which can aid in weight loss efforts by enhancing overall mobility and endurance.

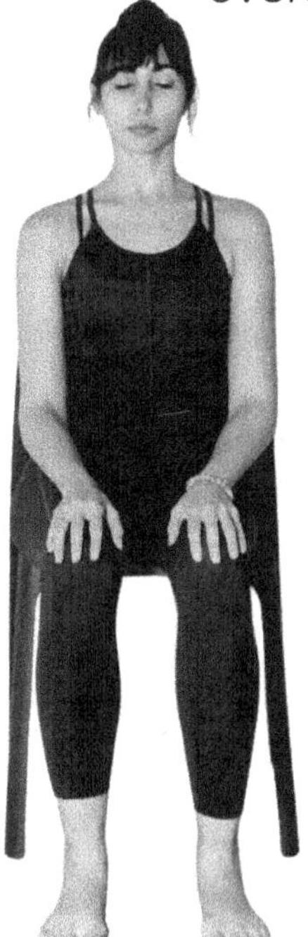 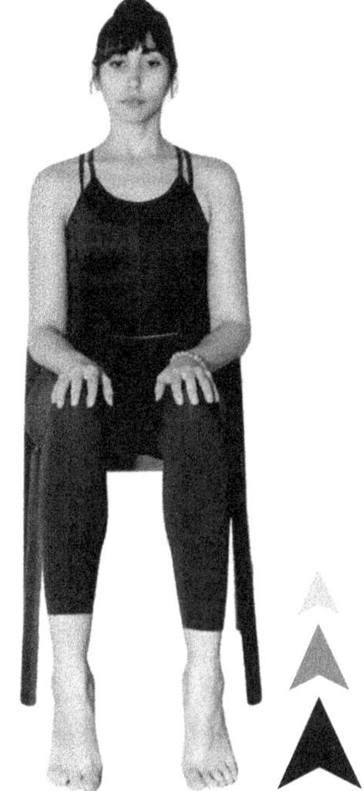

## PREPARATION

- Sit in a sturdy, armless chair with your back straight and feet flat on the floor, hip-width apart.
- Rest your hands on your thighs or the sides of the chair for balance.
- Ensure your posture is upright, with your shoulders relaxed and your core engaged.

## EXECUTION

1. Slowly lift your heels off the floor as high as you can, keeping the balls of your feet and toes on the ground.
2. Pause at the top of the movement for a count of 2-3 seconds, feeling the contraction in your calf muscles.
3. Gradually lower your heels back down to the floor, controlling the movement to maximize muscle engagement.
4. Aim for 10-15 repetitions, gradually increasing the number of sets as your strength improves.

### Tips and Advice to Avoid Common Mistakes

If you experience any discomfort in your feet or ankles, reduce the range of motion or the number of repetitions.

# Seated Toe Taps

**PURPOSE:** To engage and strengthen the core muscles, improve lower body circulation, and enhance coordination and balance from a seated position.

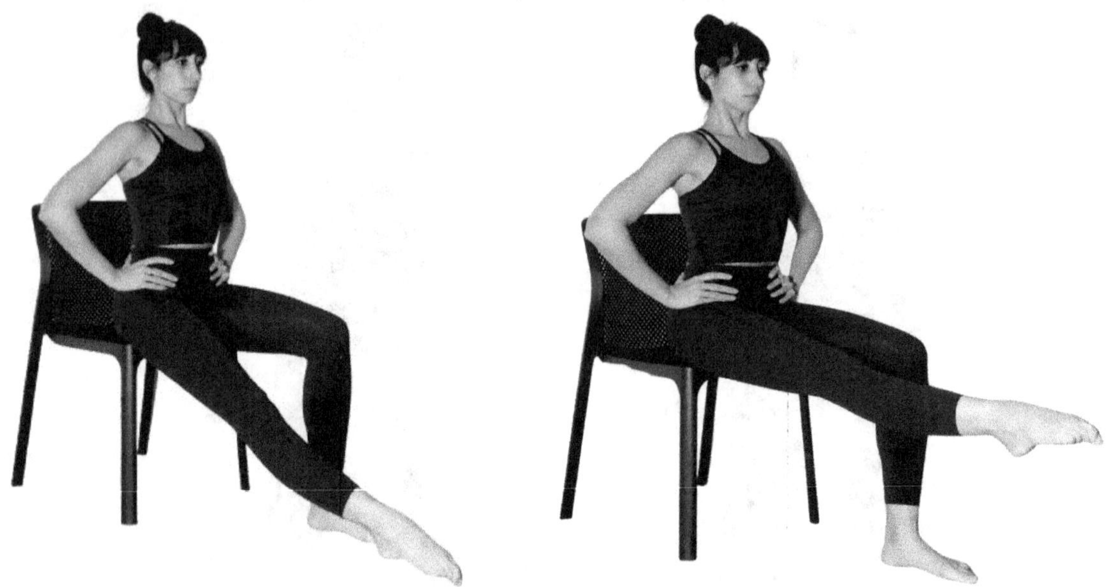

## PREPARATION

- Sit on the edge of a sturdy, armless chair with your feet flat on the ground, hip-width apart.
- Keep your back straight and engage your core by pulling your belly button towards your spine.
- Place your hands on your hips or rest them on the sides of the chair for stability.

## EXECUTION

1. Lift your right foot a few inches off the floor, keeping your leg straight.
2. Tap the floor lightly with your toes, then lift your foot back to the starting position.
3. Repeat this tapping motion for 10-15 repetitions, maintaining a controlled and steady pace.
4. Switch to your left foot and perform the same number of repetitions.
5. Aim to complete 2-3 sets on each leg, focusing on the precision of the movement rather than speed.

### Tips and Advice to Avoid Common Mistakes

Keep your shoulders down and relaxed throughout the exercise to avoid creating tension in the neck and upper back.

# Seated Balance Hold

**PURPOSE:** To enhance core stability and balance while seated, which is crucial for improving posture and reducing the risk of falls.

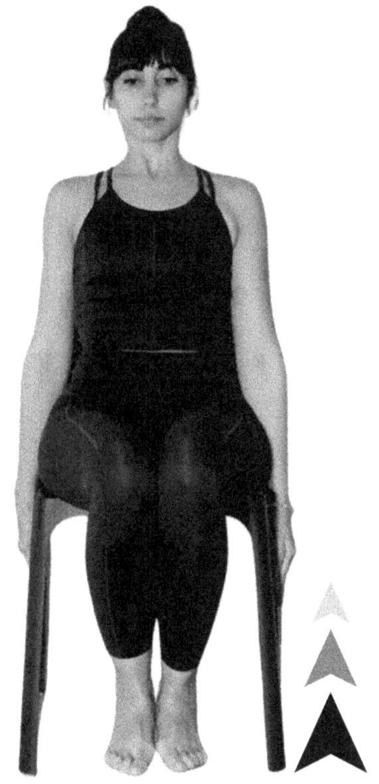

## PREPARATION

- Select a stable chair without wheels and sit at the edge with your feet flat on the floor, hip-width apart.
- Place your hands on your thighs or the sides of the chair for support.
- Sit up tall, engaging your abdominal muscles slightly to create a straight line from your head to your tailbone.

## EXECUTION

1. Gently lift both feet off the floor, keeping your knees bent. You will balance on your sit bones with your legs in the air.
2. Hold this position while you take 3-5 deep breaths, focusing on keeping your core engaged and your spine straight.
3. Slowly lower your feet back to the ground and relax your core muscles.
4. Repeat the exercise 5-10 times, depending on your comfort level and ability to maintain good form.

**Tips and Advice to Avoid Common Mistakes**

Keep your movements slow and controlled to prevent any strain on your lower back.

# Upper Body Strength and Flexibility

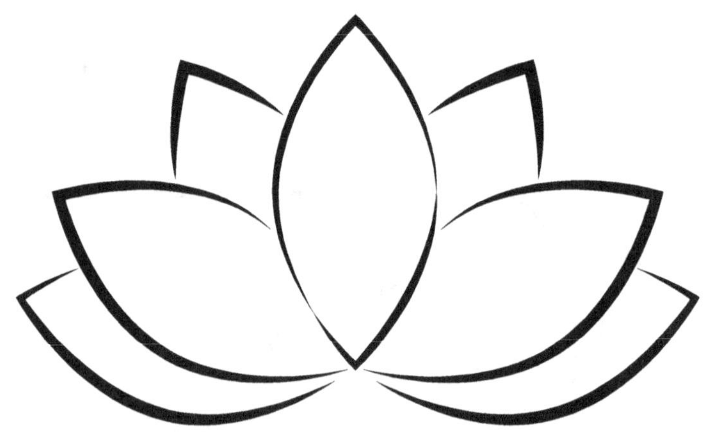

**Scan the QR code to view the 10 exercises included in this section.**

# Seated Shoulder Rolls

**PURPOSE:** To increase flexibility and reduce tension in the shoulders and upper back, promoting better posture and aiding in the overall weight loss process by encouraging a more active and pain-free range of motion.

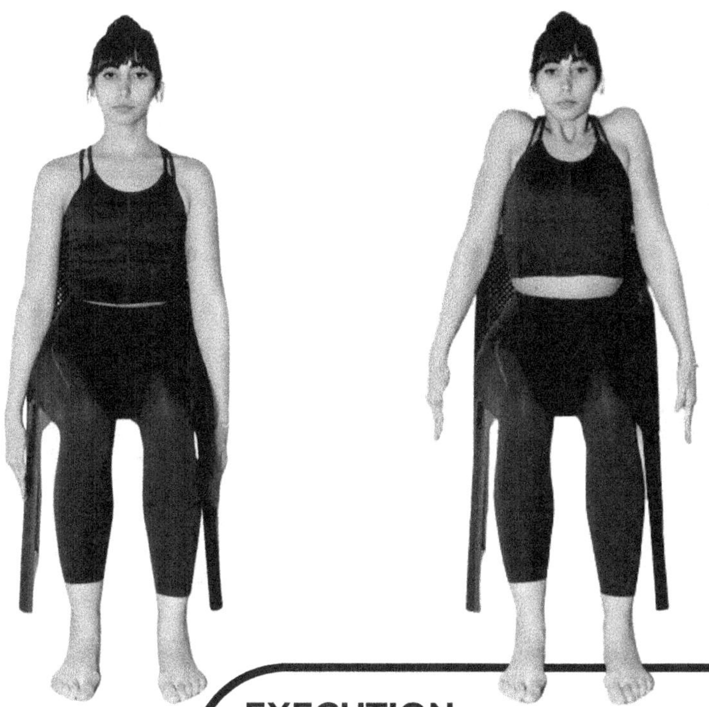

## PREPARATION

- Sit in a sturdy, armless chair with your feet flat on the floor, hip-width apart.
- Keep your back straight, engaging your core slightly to support your spine.
- Relax your arms down by your sides, allowing your hands to rest gently on your thighs or lap.

## EXECUTION

1. Inhale deeply and slowly lift your shoulders towards your ears, aiming for a smooth, controlled movement.
2. Exhale and gently roll your shoulders back, drawing them down to create a circular motion.
3. Continue this rolling motion for 5-10 repetitions, focusing on the sensation of releasing tension with each roll.
4. After completing the backward rolls, reverse the direction: inhale to lift your shoulders towards your ears, then exhale and roll them forward, again performing 5-10 repetitions.
5. Throughout the exercise, maintain a steady, rhythmic breathing pattern to enhance relaxation and effectiveness of the movement.

# Seated Arm Raises

**PURPOSE:** To strengthen the shoulders and upper back, improve posture, and enhance flexibility.

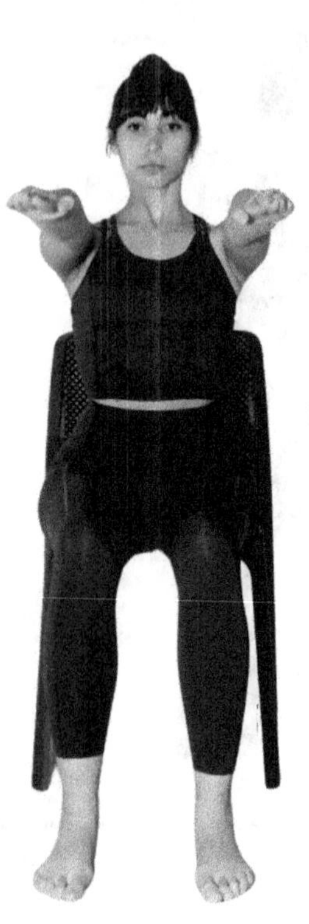

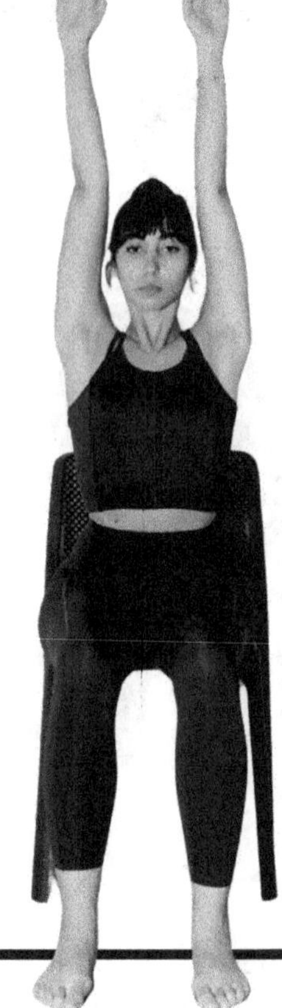

## PREPARATION

- Sit in a sturdy, armless chair with your feet flat on the ground, hip-width apart.
- Keep your back straight and engage your core muscles to support your spine.
- Relax your shoulders down away from your ears to start in a neutral position.

## EXECUTION

1. Extend your arms straight out in front of you at shoulder height, palms facing down.
2. Keeping your arms straight, slowly raise them up overhead, aiming to bring your biceps close to your ears, without shrugging your shoulders.
3. Pause briefly at the top of the movement, ensuring your shoulders remain relaxed and away from your ears.
4. Slowly lower your arms back to the starting position in front of you at shoulder height.
5. Perform 10-15 repetitions, focusing on smooth, controlled movements throughout the exercise.

# Seated Chest Opener

**PURPOSE:** To open the chest and shoulders, improving posture and breathing capacity.

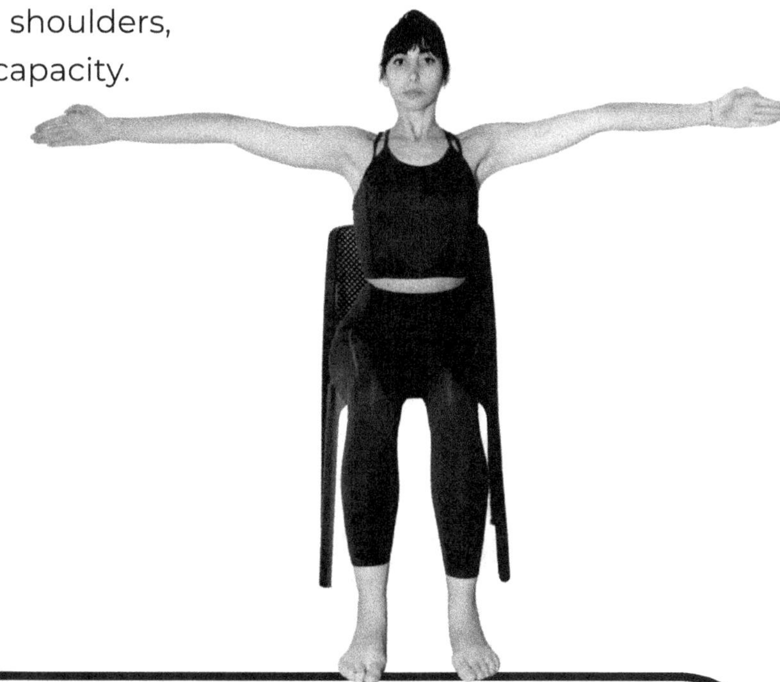

## PREPARATION

- Sit in a sturdy, armless chair with your feet flat on the floor, hip-width apart.
- Keep your back straight, engaging your core slightly to support your spine.
- Relax your arms down by your sides, allowing your hands to rest gently on your thighs or lap.

## EXECUTION

1. Inhale deeply and slowly lift your shoulders towards your ears, aiming for a smooth, controlled movement.
2. Exhale and gently roll your shoulders back, drawing them down to create a circular motion.
3. Continue this rolling motion for 5-10 repetitions, focusing on the sensation of releasing tension with each roll.
4. After completing the backward rolls, reverse the direction: inhale to lift your shoulders towards your ears, then exhale and roll them forward, again performing 5-10 repetitions.
5. Throughout the exercise, maintain a steady, rhythmic breathing pattern to enhance relaxation and effectiveness of the movement.

### Tips and Advice to Avoid Common Mistakes

Ensure that the movement is coming from your shoulders and not your neck to avoid straining the neck muscles.

# Seated Tricep Stretch

**PURPOSE:** To stretch and strengthen the triceps muscles, which are located on the back of the upper arms.

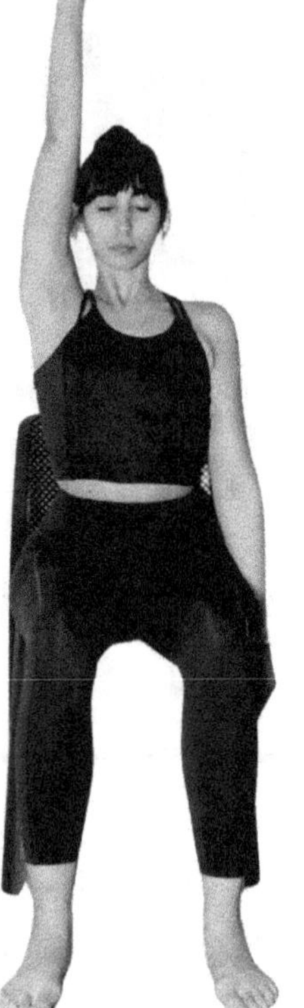 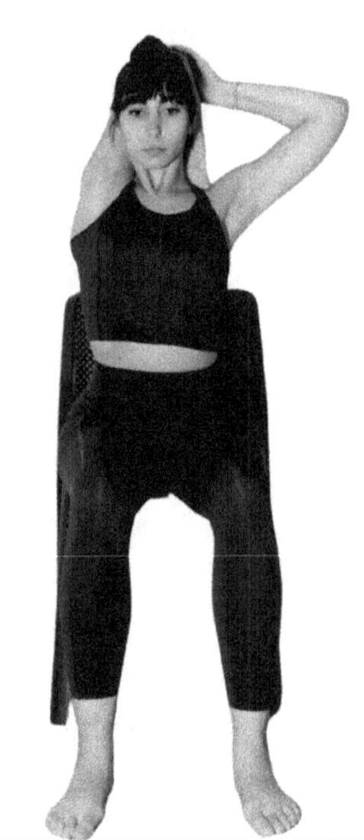

## PREPARATION
- Sit in a sturdy, armless chair with your feet planted firmly on the ground, hip-width apart.
- Keep your back straight and engage your core to support your spine.
- Raise your right arm towards the ceiling, keeping your shoulder down away from your ear.

## EXECUTION
1. Bend your right elbow, bringing your right hand down towards the middle of your back, palm facing your back. Aim to reach as far down your spine as comfortably possible.
2. Place your left hand on your right elbow to gently deepen the stretch without forcing it.
3. Keep your head upright and your gaze forward, ensuring you do not strain your neck.
4. Hold this position for 15-30 seconds, focusing on a deep stretch in your right tricep.
5. Slowly release your hands and return to the starting position.
6. Repeat the stretch with your left arm, switching the roles of your hands.

# Seated Shoulder Blade Squeeze

**PURPOSE:** To strengthen the muscles between the shoulder blades, improve posture, and reduce tension in the upper back and neck.

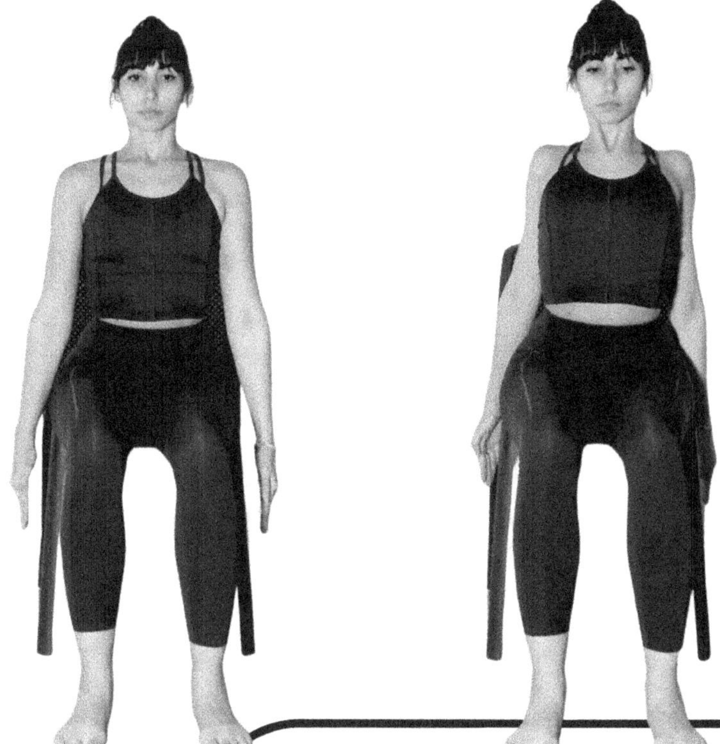

## PREPARATION

- Sit in a sturdy, armless chair with your feet flat on the floor, hip-width apart.
- Keep your back straight, shoulders relaxed, and gaze forward.
- Place your hands on your thighs or let them hang by your sides.

## EXECUTION

1. Inhale deeply and, as you exhale, gently draw your shoulder blades towards each other, as if trying to hold a pencil between them.
2. Keep your neck long and shoulders down, away from your ears, to avoid creating tension.
3. Hold the squeeze for 3-5 seconds, focusing on the engagement between your shoulder blades.
4. Slowly release the squeeze and return to your starting position with a controlled movement.
5. Repeat the exercise 10-15 times, ensuring smooth and deliberate movements throughout.

### Tips and Advice to Avoid Common Mistakes

Start with gentle squeezes and gradually increase the intensity as your strength and flexibility improve, but always within a comfortable range of motion.

# Seated Arm Reach

**PURPOSE:** To increase upper body strength and flexibility, specifically targeting the shoulders, arms, and upper back.

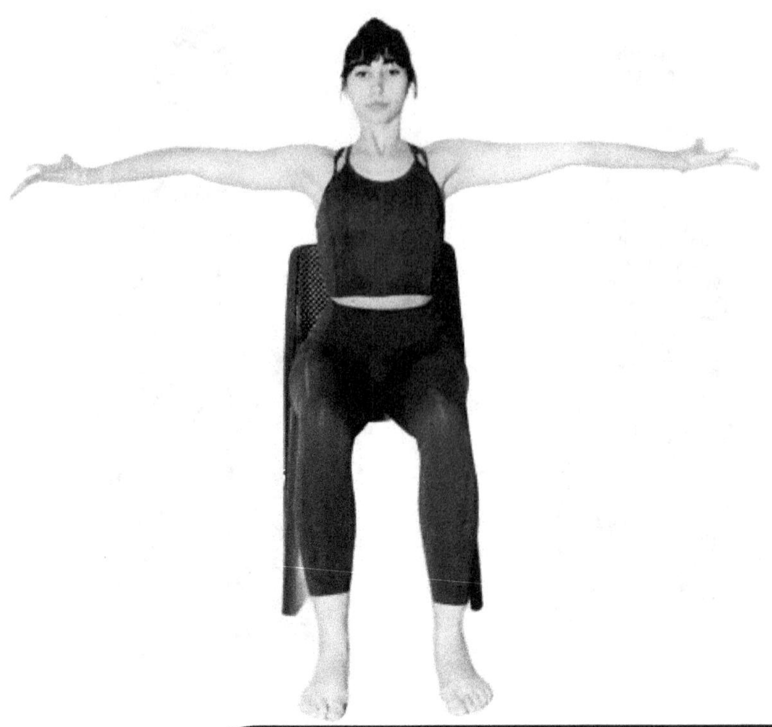

## PREPARATION

- Sit in a sturdy, armless chair with your feet flat on the floor, hip-width apart. Ensure your back is straight, and your core is engaged.
- Relax your shoulders down away from your ears, and let your arms hang loosely by your sides.

## EXECUTION

1. Inhale deeply and, as you exhale, slowly raise your arms to the side until they are parallel with the floor, palms facing down.
2. Keep your shoulders relaxed and down, avoiding any shrugging or tension in the neck area.
3. Gently turn your palms up towards the ceiling and reach through your fingertips as if trying to touch the walls on either side of the room.
4. Hold this position for a count of 5-10 seconds, focusing on the stretch and strength in your arms and shoulders.
5. Inhale and, as you exhale, slowly lower your arms back to your sides.
6. Repeat the movement 5-10 times, depending on your comfort level and ability to maintain good form.

# Seated Wrist Circles

**PURPOSE:** To improve wrist flexibility and strength, which is essential for maintaining hand and arm health.

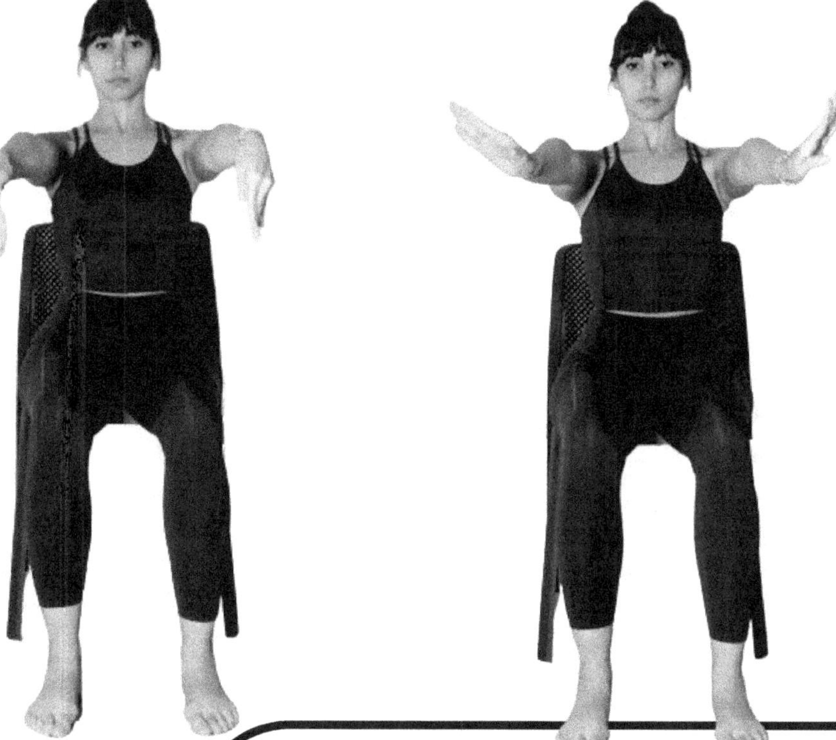

## PREPARATION

- Sit in a sturdy, armless chair with your feet flat on the ground, hip-width apart.
- Keep your back straight and shoulders relaxed.
- Extend your arms straight out in front of you, at shoulder level, with palms facing down.

## EXECUTION

1. Slowly start to rotate your wrists in a clockwise direction, making small circles.
2. Continue these circular motions for about 15-20 seconds.
3. Pause, then rotate your wrists in a counterclockwise direction for another 15-20 seconds.
4. Keep your arms steady and focus on moving only your wrists to isolate the muscles being worked.

**Tips and Advice to Avoid Common Mistakes**

Keep your arms extended but not locked at the elbows to maintain a slight bend, which helps prevent joint stress.

# Seated Neck Stretch

**PURPOSE:** To relieve tension in the neck and shoulders, improve flexibility, and enhance circulation in the upper body.

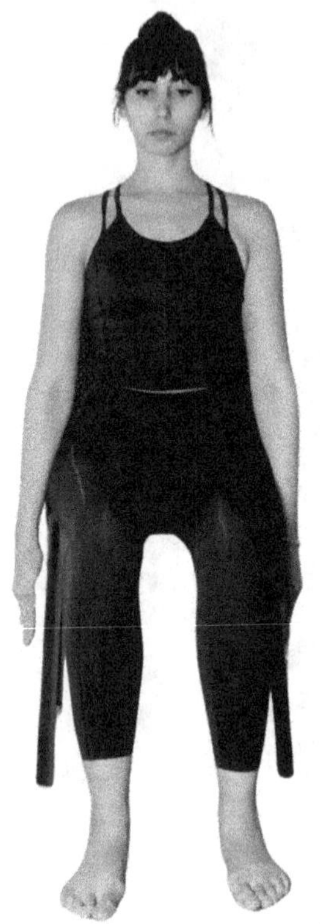 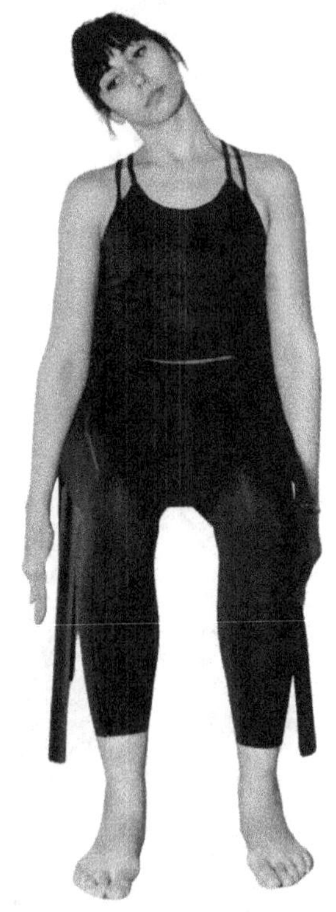

## PREPARATION

- Sit in a sturdy, armless chair with your feet flat on the ground, hip-width apart.
- Keep your back straight and shoulders relaxed, resting your hands on your thighs or the sides of the chair.
- Take a few deep breaths to center yourself and prepare for the stretch.

## EXECUTION

1. Gently lower your right ear towards your right shoulder, keeping your left shoulder relaxed and avoiding lifting it towards your ear.
2. Hold the stretch for 20-30 seconds, breathing deeply and allowing the muscles on the left side of your neck to elongate.
3. Slowly lift your head back to the center and repeat the stretch on the left side, lowering your left ear towards your left shoulder.
4. After holding the stretch on the left side, return your head to the center position.
5. For an additional stretch, gently turn your head to look over your right shoulder, holding for 20-30 seconds, then repeat on the left side.
6. Complete 2-3 repetitions of each stretch on both sides.

# Seated Upper Back Stretch

**PURPOSE:** To stretch and relieve tension in the upper back and shoulder area, improving flexibility and posture.

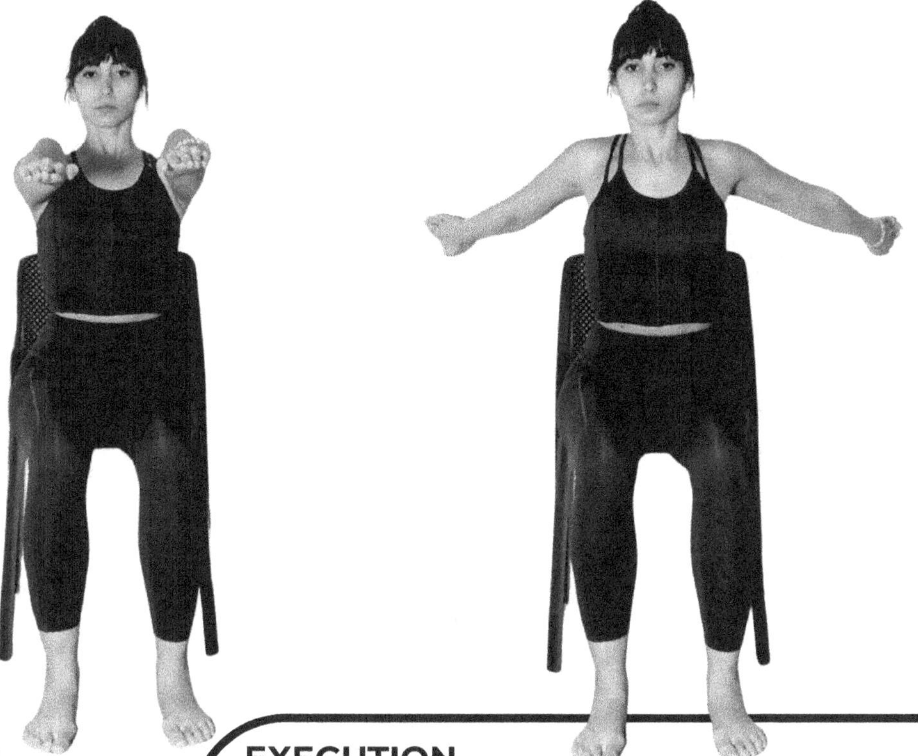

## PREPARATION

- Sit in a sturdy, armless chair with your feet flat on the ground, hip-width apart.
- Keep your back straight and shoulders relaxed, aligning your ears over your shoulders.
- Place your hands on your lap or by your sides.

## EXECUTION

1. Extend your arms straight in front of you at shoulder height, palms facing down.
2. Slowly move your arms apart, bringing them as far back as they can go while squeezing your shoulder blades together. Imagine you are trying to hold a pencil between your shoulder blades.
3. Keep your neck straight and chin slightly tucked, ensuring your gaze is forward and not straining upwards or downwards.
4. Hold this position for 15-30 seconds, taking deep breaths to help deepen the stretch.
5. Gently release your arms back to the starting position in front of you.
6. Repeat the stretch 2-3 times, resting briefly between repetitions.

# Seated Side Arm Stretch



**PURPOSE:** To stretch and strengthen the muscles along the sides of your torso, improving flexibility and aiding in the reduction of waistline fat.

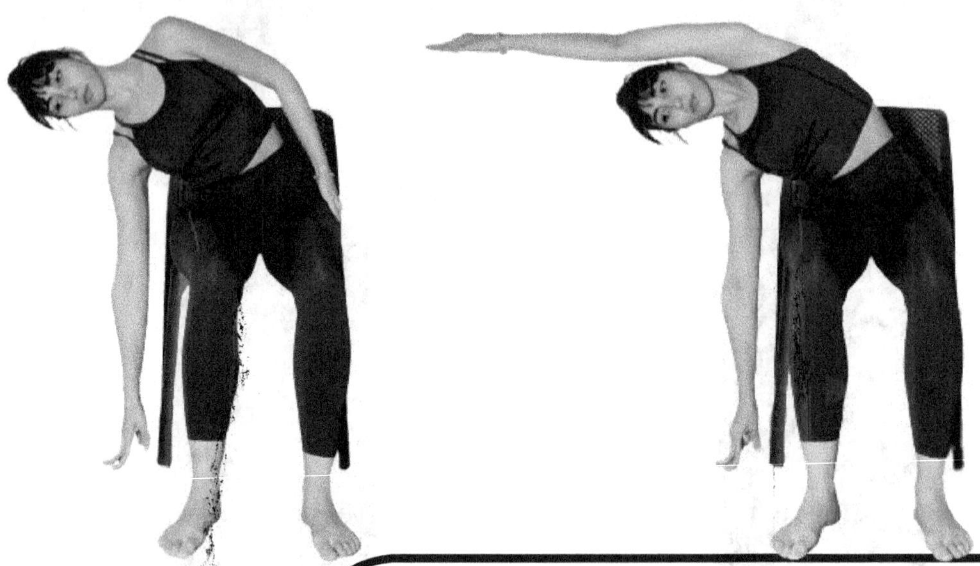

## PREPARATION

- Sit upright in a sturdy chair without arms, feet flat on the ground, and knees aligned over your ankles.
- Place your hands on the sides of the chair seat for stability.
- Engage your core muscles gently to support your spine.

## EXECUTION

1. Inhale deeply, and as you exhale, slowly lean your torso to the right, sliding your right hand down the side of the chair towards the floor.
2. Keep your left buttock firmly in contact with the chair seat to ensure both hips remain squared and grounded.
3. Extend your left arm up over your head, creating a straight line from your left fingertips down to your left hip, enhancing the side stretch.
4. Hold this position for 3-5 breaths, focusing on elongating your torso with each inhalation and deepening the stretch with each exhalation.
5. Inhale as you gently return to the starting position, bringing your left hand back to the side of the chair.
6. Repeat the stretch on the opposite side, sliding your left hand down the chair as you lean to the left and extending your right arm overhead.
7. Perform 3-5 repetitions on each side, alternating smoothly and maintaining controlled breathing throughout.

# Lower Body Strength and Mobility

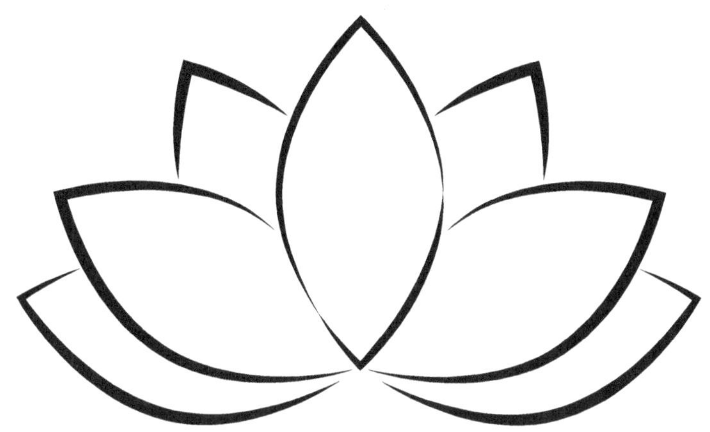

Scan the QR code to view the 10 exercises included in this section.

# Seated Ankle Circles

**PURPOSE:** To improve ankle flexibility and circulation, which is essential for maintaining mobility and reducing the risk of falls.

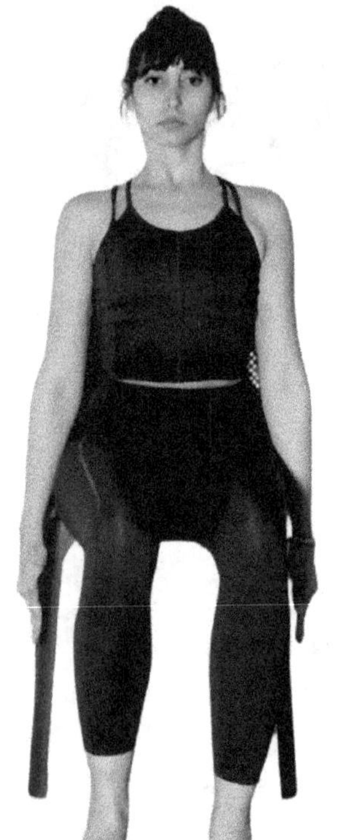 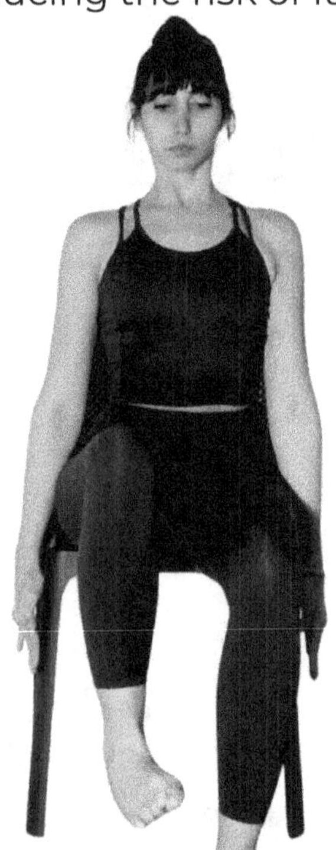

## PREPARATION

- Sit in a sturdy, armless chair with a straight back to ensure proper posture.
- Place your feet flat on the floor, hip-width apart.
- Keep your back straight, shoulders relaxed, and hands resting on your thighs or the sides of the chair for balance.

## EXECUTION

1. Lift your right foot off the floor slightly, keeping your leg bent at the knee.
2. Begin to rotate your right ankle slowly, making clockwise circles. Aim for smooth, controlled movements.
3. Continue the clockwise circles for 15-20 seconds, then switch directions, making counterclockwise circles for another 15-20 seconds.
4. Gently place your right foot back on the ground and repeat the exercise with your left ankle, following the same duration and directions for the circles.

### Tips and Advice to Avoid Common Mistakes

Ensure that the movement comes from the ankle, not the whole leg. The focus should be on isolating the ankle to maximize flexibility and strength in that area.

# Seated Warrior Pose Sequence

**PURPOSE:** To build strength and flexibility in the legs, open the hips, and improve balance while stretching the upper body.

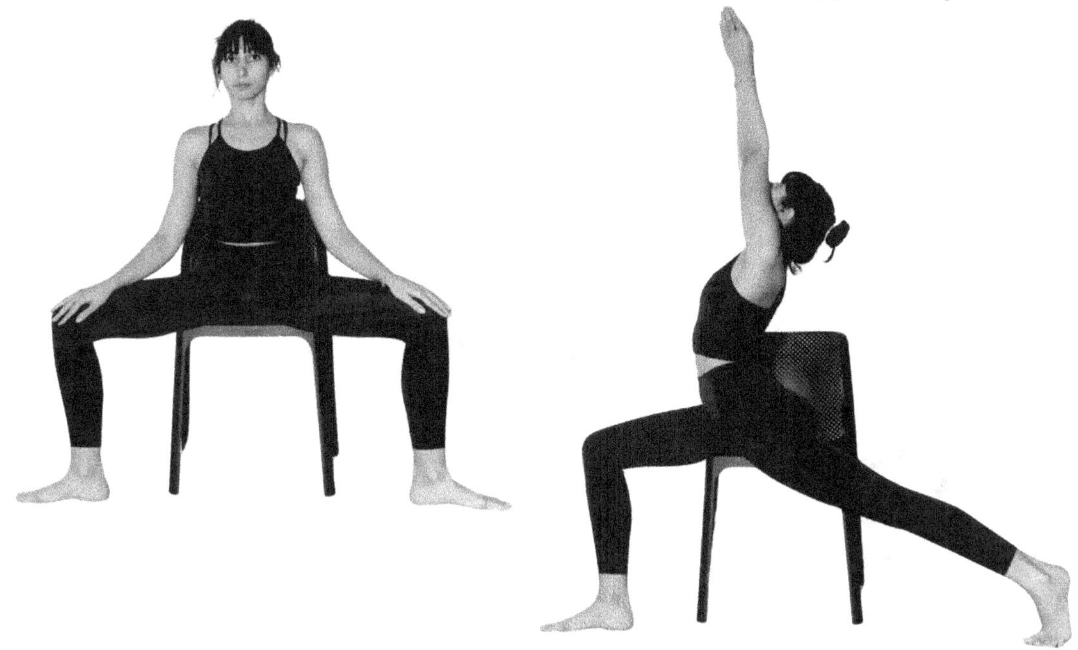

## PREPARATION

- Sit comfortably at the edge of a sturdy chair, keeping your back straight and feet flat on the floor.
- Ensure there is enough space to extend one leg behind the chair during the exercise.

## EXECUTION

1. Sit upright with your hands resting on your thighs. Take a deep breath to center yourself.
2. Spread your legs wide with your feet firmly planted on the floor. Place your hands on your thighs for support, keeping your back straight.
3. Slide your right leg backward, extending it behind you with your toes pointed forward. Keep your left knee bent at a 90-degree angle and your left foot flat on the ground. Rest your hands lightly on your left thigh for balance.
4. Raise both arms above your head with your palms facing each other. Keep your torso upright and feel the stretch along your arms and back. Hold the position for a few breaths.
5. Lower your arms, bringing your palms together in a prayer position at your chest. Breathe deeply and hold the position. Then, return to the starting position and repeat the steps on the opposite side.

# Seated Hamstring Stretch

**PURPOSE:** To improve ankle flexibility and circulation, which is essential for maintaining mobility and reducing the risk of falls.

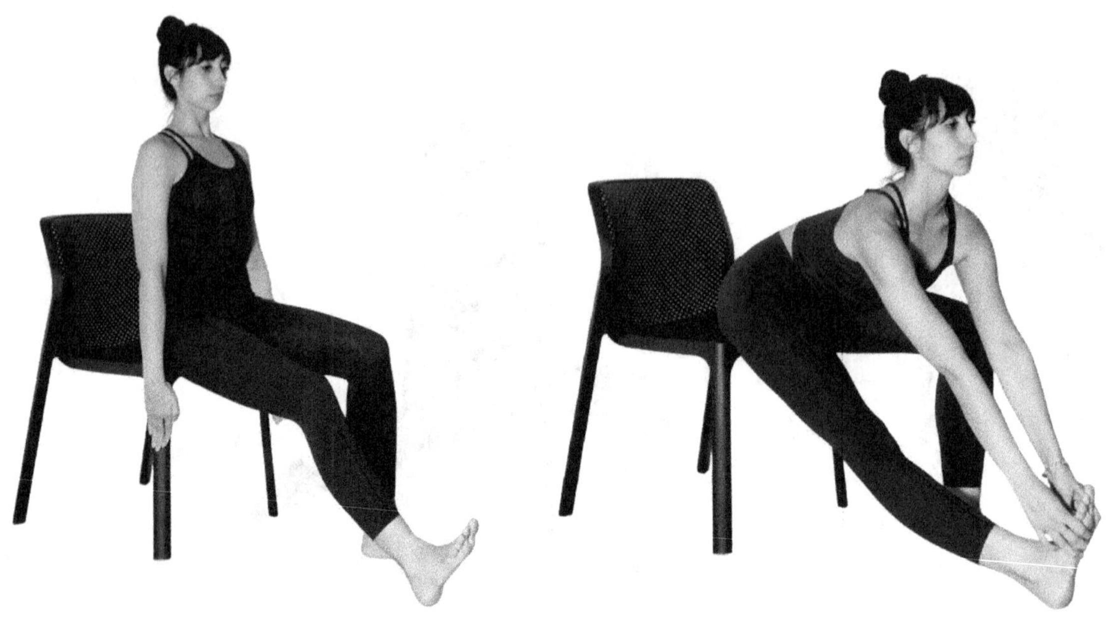

## PREPARATION

- Sit on the edge of a sturdy, armless chair with both feet flat on the floor, hip-width apart.
- Keep your back straight, engaging your core muscles to support your spine.
- Place your hands on your thighs for added stability.

## EXECUTION

1. Extend your right leg straight in front of you, resting your heel on the floor with your toes pointed upwards.
2. Keep your left foot flat on the ground, maintaining a slight bend in your left knee.
3. Inhale deeply, and as you exhale, gently hinge forward at the hips, keeping your back straight, and reach towards your right toes with your hands.
4. Go only as far as comfortable without rounding your back, aiming to feel a gentle stretch along the back of your right thigh.
5. Hold this position for 15-30 seconds, taking deep breaths to help deepen the stretch.
6. Slowly return to the starting position and repeat the stretch on the left leg.

# Seated Quad Stretch

**PURPOSE:** To stretch and strengthen the quadriceps muscles, which are crucial for knee stability and overall mobility.

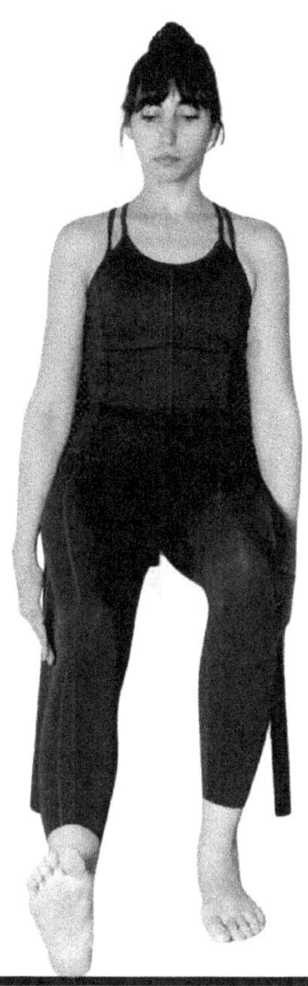

## PREPARATION

- Sit in a sturdy, armless chair with your feet flat on the ground and knees bent at a 90-degree angle.
- Keep your back straight and engage your core to support your upper body.
- Place your hands on the sides of the chair or on your lap for balance.

## EXECUTION

1. Extend one leg out in front of you, keeping the other foot on the ground.
2. Flex your foot (the one being extended) towards you, aiming to straighten the leg as much as possible without locking the knee.
3. Hold this position for 15-30 seconds, focusing on feeling the stretch along the back of your thigh.
4. Slowly lower the leg back to the starting position.
5. Repeat the stretch with the other leg.
6. Aim for 2-3 repetitions on each leg.

### Tips and Advice to Avoid Common Mistakes

If you experience any discomfort in your feet or ankles, reduce the range of motion or the number of repetitions.

# Seated Hip Flexor Stretch

**PURPOSE:** To stretch the hip flexors, which can become tight from prolonged periods of sitting.

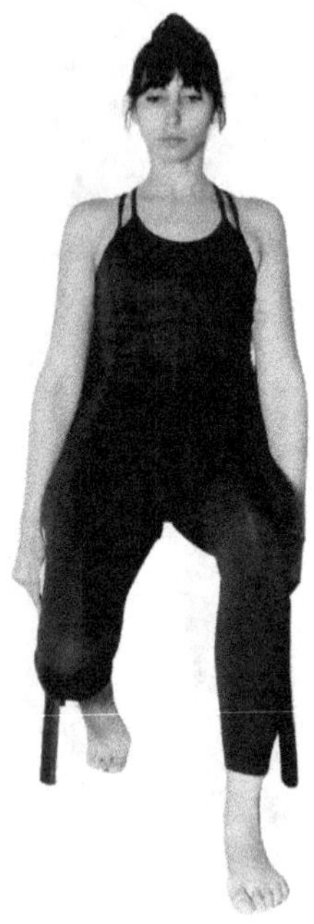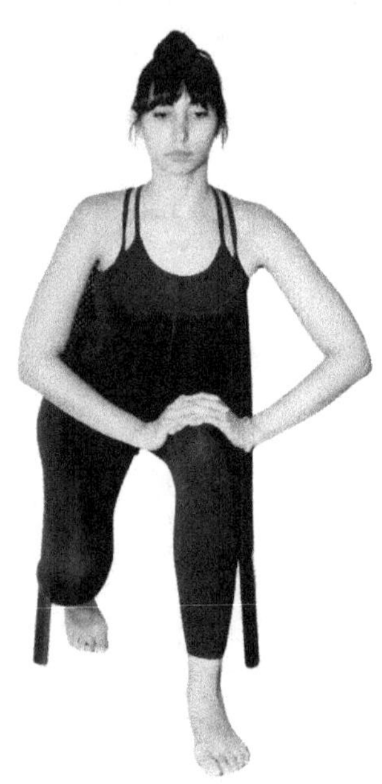

## PREPARATION

- Sit towards the front of a sturdy, armless chair with your feet flat on the ground, hip-width apart.
- Keep your back straight, engaging your core muscles to support your spine.
- Shift slightly to the edge of the chair to allow for greater range of motion during the stretch.

## EXECUTION

1. Gently extend your right leg back, placing the ball of your foot on the ground and keeping your heel lifted. If necessary, scoot further towards the edge of the chair to achieve this position comfortably.
2. Ensure your left foot remains flat on the floor, directly under your left knee, forming a 90-degree angle.
3. Place your hands on your left thigh for stability, keeping your shoulders relaxed and your spine straight.
4. Gradually lean forward from your hips, pushing slightly into your left thigh while keeping your back straight, to intensify the stretch in your right hip flexor.
5. Hold this position for 20-30 seconds, breathing deeply and focusing on relaxing the hip muscles.
6. Slowly return to the starting position and switch legs, repeating the stretch on the left side.

# Seated Glute Squeeze

**PURPOSE:** To strengthen the gluteal muscles, which are essential for stability, mobility, and overall lower body strength.

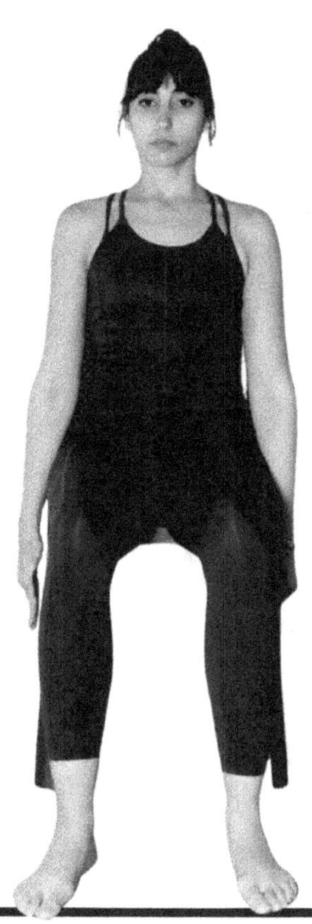

## PREPARATION

- Sit in a sturdy, armless chair with your feet flat on the ground, hip-width apart.
- Keep your back straight and engage your core to support your upper body.
- Place your hands on the sides of the chair for stability.

## EXECUTION

1. Squeeze your glutes as tightly as you can, imagining you are trying to hold a coin between your cheeks.
2. Hold the squeeze for 3-5 seconds, focusing on the contraction in your gluteal muscles.
3. Slowly release the squeeze, allowing your muscles to relax fully.
4. Repeat the exercise 10-15 times, ensuring you maintain the intensity of the squeeze each time.

**Tips and Advice to Avoid Common Mistakes**

Ensure you are only squeezing your glutes and not tensing your entire body. Keep your shoulders relaxed and your breathing steady.

# Seated Inner Thigh Squeeze

**PURPOSE:** To strengthen the inner thigh muscles, which are crucial for stabilizing your pelvis and supporting your spine.

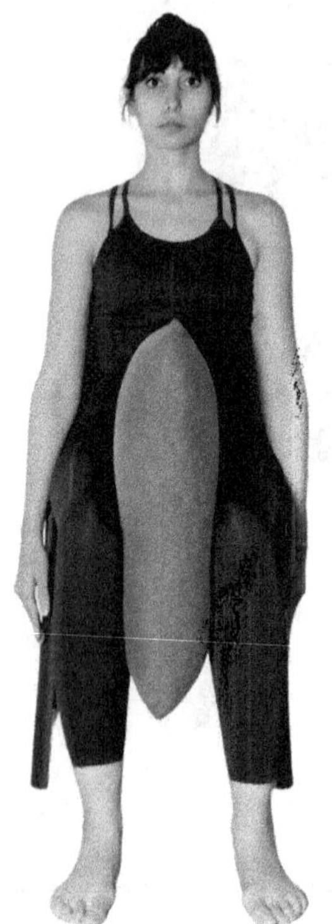 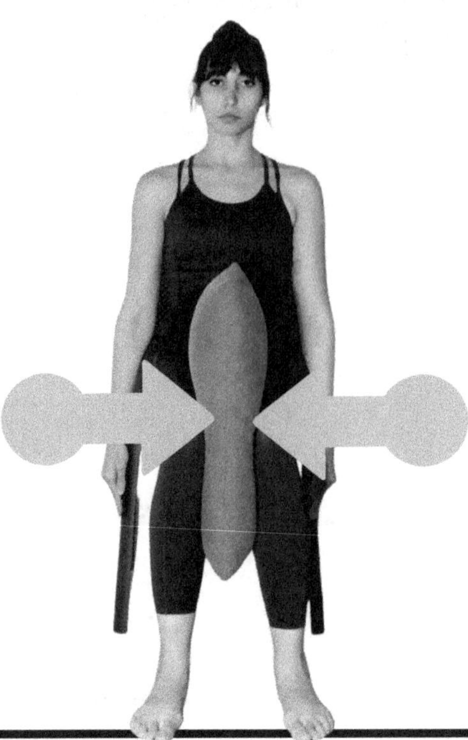

## PREPARATION

- Sit in a sturdy, armless chair with your feet flat on the floor, hip-width apart.
- Keep your back straight, engaging your core to support your upright posture.
- Place a soft, medium-sized ball (like a Pilates ball or even a thick pillow) between your knees.

## EXECUTION

1. With the ball securely in place, slowly squeeze your knees together, applying pressure to the ball.
2. Hold the squeeze for 3-5 seconds, focusing on engaging the muscles in your inner thighs.
3. Gradually release the pressure, allowing the ball to return to its original shape without losing contact between your knees.
4. Repeat the squeeze and release motion for 10-15 repetitions, ensuring smooth and controlled movements throughout the exercise.

## Tips and Advice to Avoid Common Mistakes

To ensure maximum benefit and minimize the risk of injury, focus on quality over quantity. It's better to perform fewer repetitions with correct form than to rush through the exercise.

# Seated Outer Thigh Lift

**PURPOSE:** To strengthen the muscles on the sides of the hips and thighs, improve balance, and enhance core stability, which is crucial for maintaining mobility and supporting weight loss efforts through increased muscle engagement.

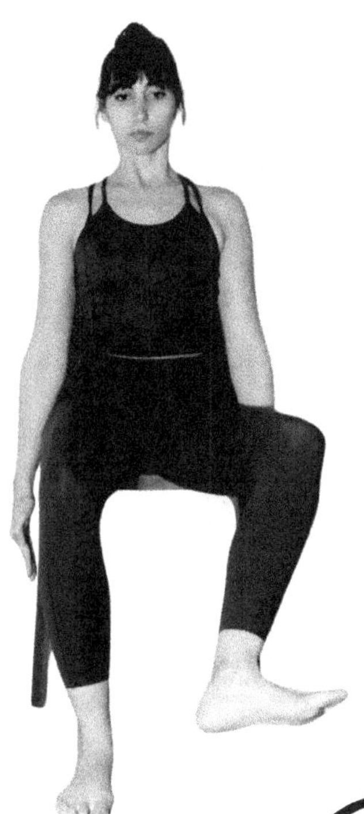 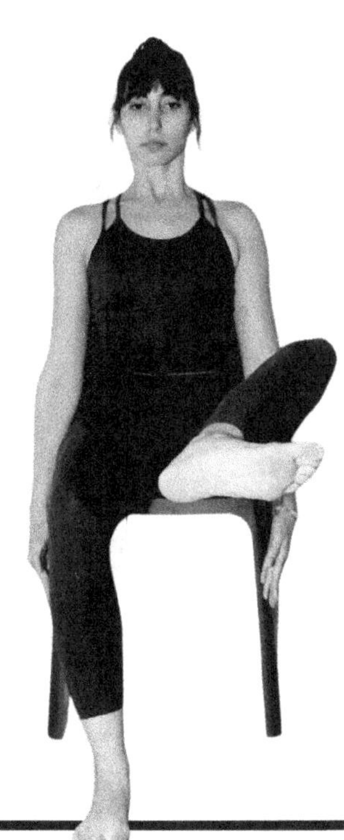

## PREPARATION

- Sit in a sturdy, armless chair with your back straight and feet flat on the floor, spaced hip-width apart.
- Engage your core by gently pulling your belly button towards your spine to provide support for your lower back.
- Place your hands on the sides of the chair seat or on your thighs for balance.

## EXECUTION

1. Shift your weight slightly to your right side, keeping your right foot firmly on the ground.
2. Slowly lift your left leg to the side, keeping the leg straight but not locked at the knee.
3. Lift the leg as high as comfortably possible without tilting your torso to the side; aim for a height where you can maintain balance and form.
4. Hold the lift for 2-3 seconds, then slowly lower your leg back to the starting position.
5. Perform 10-15 repetitions on the left side before switching to lift your right leg in the same manner.
6. Aim to complete 2-3 sets on each side, depending on your comfort and ability.

# Seated Ankle Pumps

**PURPOSE:** To improve circulation in the lower legs and feet, enhance ankle flexibility, and reduce swelling.

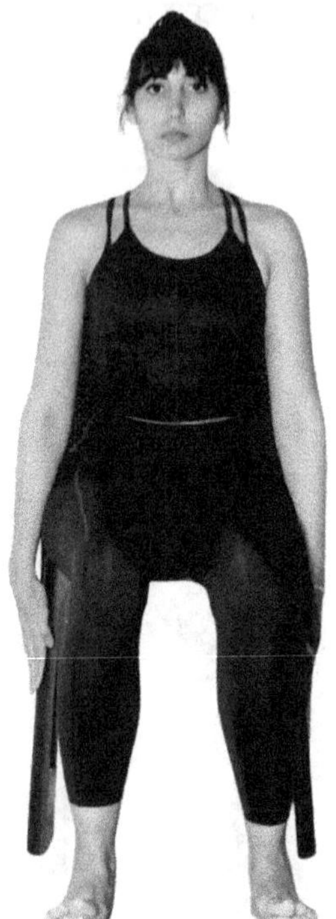 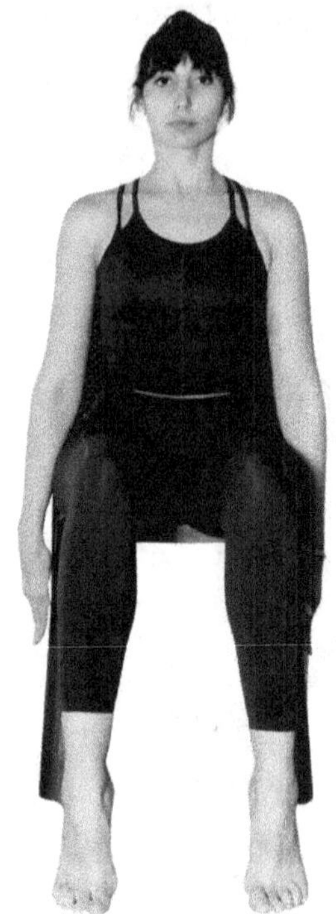

## PREPARATION

- Sit in a sturdy, armless chair with a straight back to support your posture.
- Place your feet flat on the floor, hip-width apart.
- Keep your back straight, shoulders relaxed, and hands resting on your thighs or the sides of the chair.

## EXECUTION

1. Lift your heels off the floor as high as you can, keeping the balls of your feet and toes on the ground.
2. Hold this position for a count of 2-3 seconds.
3. Slowly lower your heels back to the floor.
4. Next, lift your toes and the balls of your feet off the ground, keeping your heels on the floor.
5. Hold this position for a count of 2-3 seconds.
6. Lower your toes and the balls of your feet back to the floor.
7. This completes one repetition. Perform 10-15 repetitions, focusing on smooth, controlled movements.

### Tips and Advice to Avoid Common Mistakes

Ensure your movements are slow and controlled. Rushing through the exercise can reduce its effectiveness and may lead to strain.

# Seated Toe Flex and Point

**PURPOSE:** To improve circulation in the lower legs and feet, increase ankle mobility, and strengthen the muscles in the foot and lower leg.

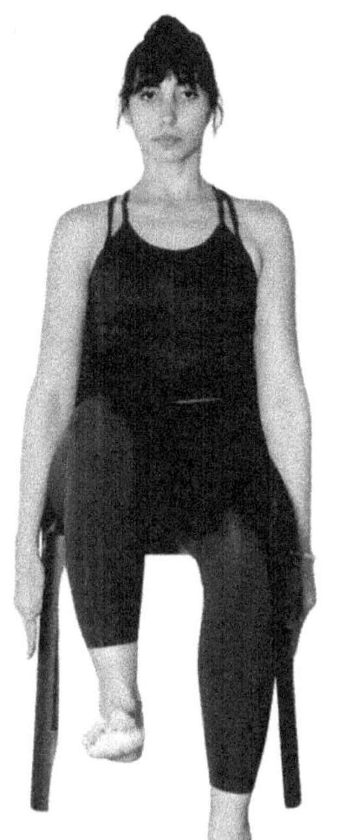 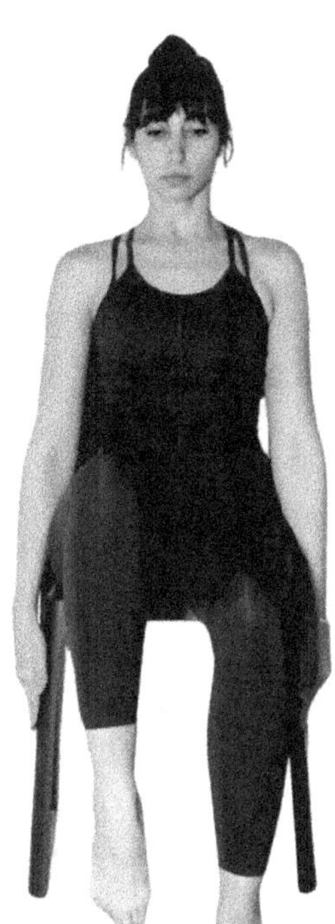

## PREPARATION

- Sit in a sturdy, armless chair with a straight back to ensure proper posture.
- Place your feet flat on the ground, hip-width apart.
- Keep your hands on your thighs or the sides of the chair for balance.

## EXECUTION

1. Lift your heels, keeping your toes on the floor, then slowly lower your heels back to the ground.
2. Lift your toes, keeping your heels on the floor, then slowly lower your toes back to the ground.
3. Continue alternating between lifting heels and toes, aiming for a smooth, controlled movement.
4. Perform this exercise for 1-2 minutes, focusing on the flexion and extension of the foot.

### Tips and Advice to Avoid Common Mistakes

Breathe evenly throughout the exercise, inhaling as you lift and exhaling as you lower, to support movement and maintain stability.

# Full-Body Movements for Fat Burning and Mobility

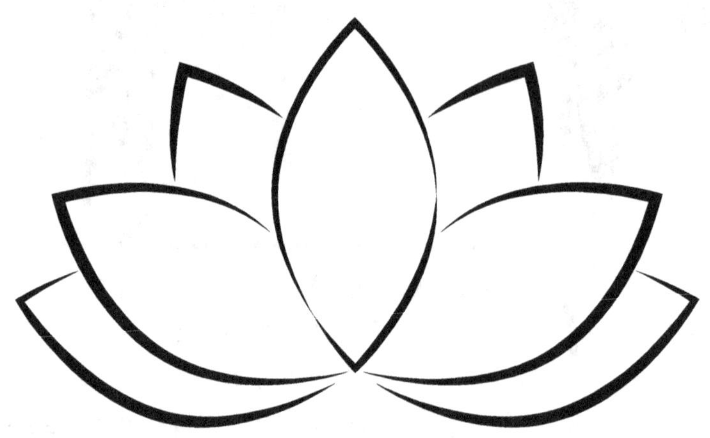

Scan the QR code to view the 12 exercises included in this section.

# Seated Full-Body Stretch

**PURPOSE:** To enhance overall flexibility and mobility by engaging multiple muscle groups simultaneously.

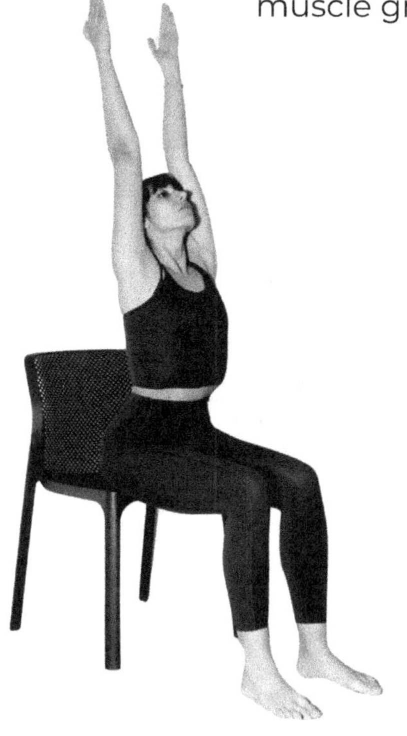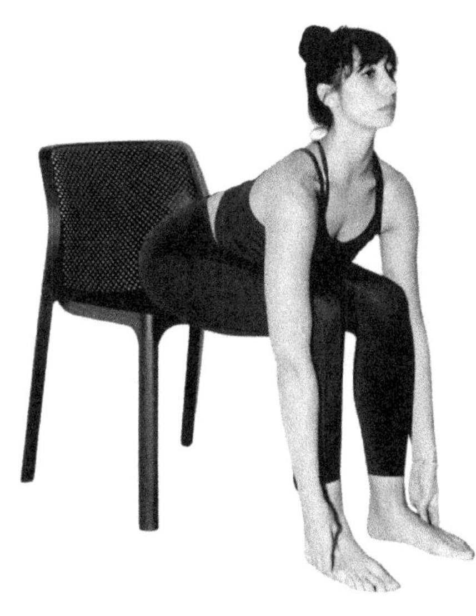

## PREPARATION

- Sit on the edge of a sturdy, armless chair with your feet planted firmly on the ground, hip-width apart.
- Keep your back straight, shoulders relaxed, and hands resting on your thighs.
- Take a few deep breaths to center yourself before beginning the exercise.

## EXECUTION

1. Inhale deeply and extend your arms overhead, reaching towards the ceiling with your fingertips.
2. As you exhale, gently hinge at the hips and lean forward, extending your hands towards your toes. Keep your back straight and neck in line with your spine.
3. Reach as far as comfortable, aiming to touch your toes or shins, depending on your flexibility.
4. Hold this forward bend for 3-5 deep breaths, feeling a stretch through your back, shoulders, and hamstrings.
5. Inhale as you slowly raise your torso back up, lifting your arms overhead once again.
6. Exhale and release your arms, lowering them back to your sides.
7. Repeat the stretch 2-3 times, focusing on smooth, fluid movements and deep breathing.

# Elevating Stretch Sequence

**PURPOSE:** To improve posture, enhance flexibility, and relieve tension in the upper body while promoting relaxation and a sense of mindfulness.

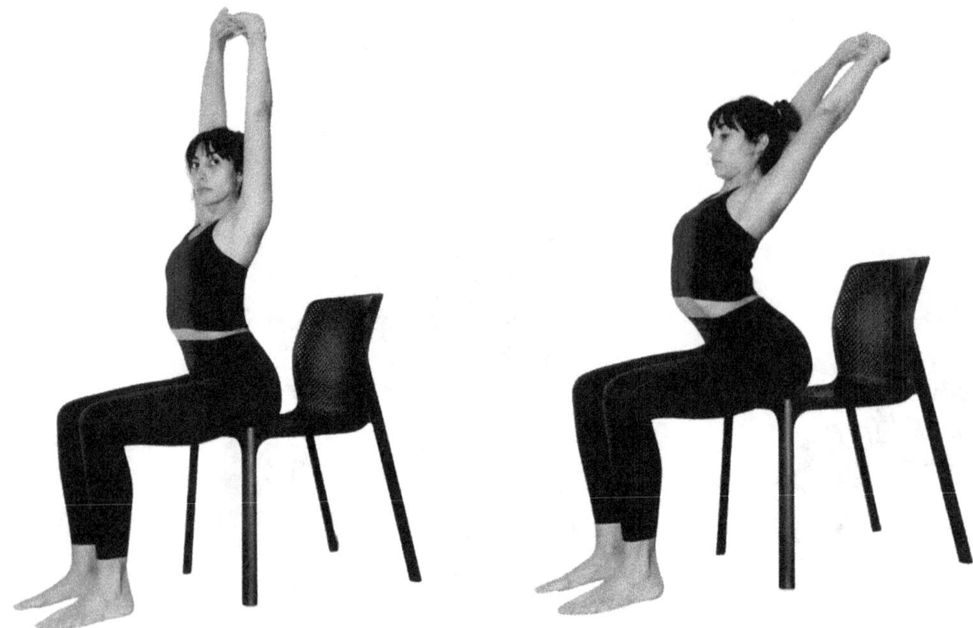

## PREPARATION
- Sit comfortably on the edge of a sturdy chair with your back straight and feet flat on the floor.
- Keep your knees bent at a 90-degree angle and your hands resting gently on your thighs.
- Take deep breath to prepare your body for movement.

## EXECUTION
1. Sit tall with your spine aligned and shoulders relaxed. Let your arms rest naturally at your sides and take a deep breath in through your nose.
2. Raise both arms above your head, interlock your fingers, and turn your palms upward. Stretch upward, feeling the lengthening along your sides. Hold for a few breaths.
3. With your arms still overhead, tilt your upper body slightly backward, opening your chest. Keep your lower back stable and avoid overextending. Breathe deeply as you feel the stretch.
4. Return to the upright position with your arms extended overhead, fingers still interlocked, and palms facing up. Hold the stretch for a few breaths.
5. Lower your arms, bringing your palms together at your chest in a prayer position. Relax your shoulders and take a few deep breaths to end the exercise.

# Chair-Assisted Squat

**PURPOSE:** To improve hip flexibility, deepen spinal twists, and enhance balance and posture while releasing tension in the lower back.

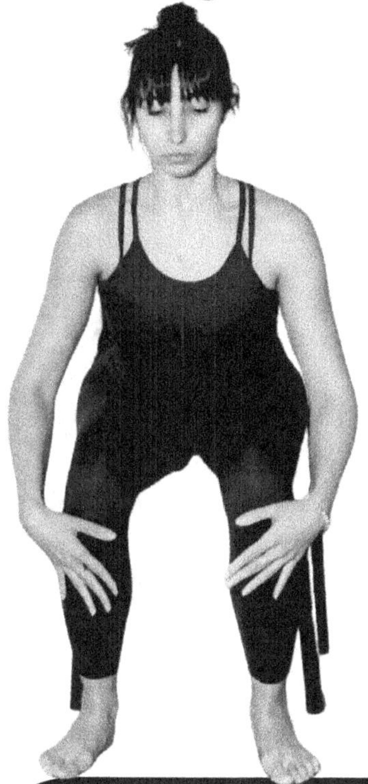

## PREPARATION

- Sit in a sturdy, armless chair with a straight back to support your posture.
- Place your feet flat on the floor, hip-width apart, ensuring your knees are aligned with your toes.
- Keep your back straight, shoulders relaxed, and bring your hands up to your chest, crossing them.

## EXECUTION

1. Inhale deeply and engage your core muscles as you lean slightly forward, keeping your back straight.
2. Slowly rise from the chair, pressing through your heels and engaging your leg muscles as you stand up.
3. Hold the standing position for a count of 2-3 seconds, focusing on your balance.
4. Carefully lower yourself back into the chair, maintaining control as you sit down.
5. This completes one repetition. Perform 10-15 repetitions, focusing on controlled movements and maintaining good posture throughout.

**Tips and Advice to Avoid Common Mistakes**

Keep your core muscles engaged throughout the exercise to maintain stability and protect your lower back.

# Seated Leg Circles

**PURPOSE:** To enhance lower body mobility and flexibility, particularly in the hips and thighs, while seated.

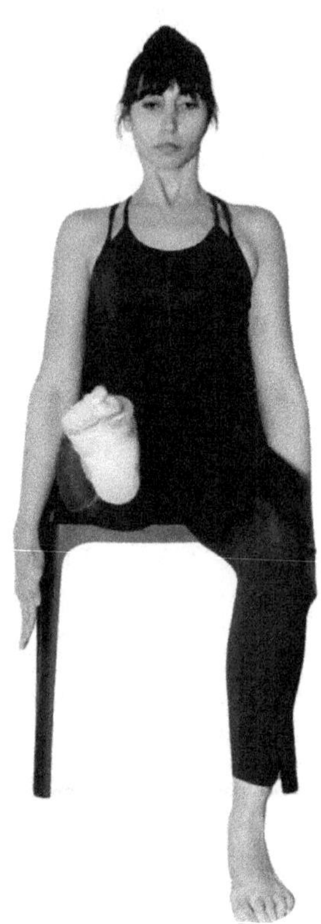 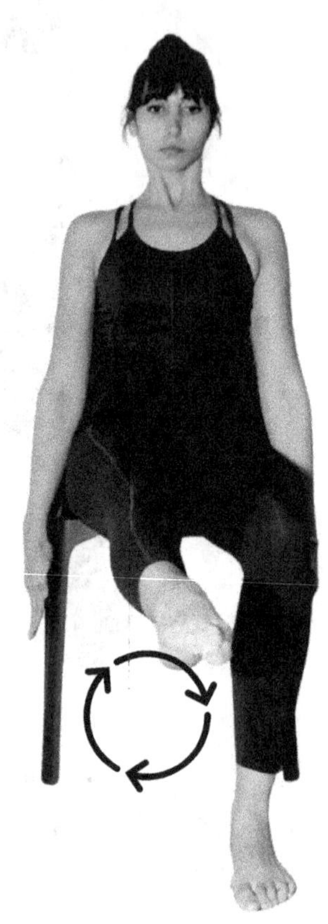

## PREPARATION

- Sit in a sturdy, armless chair with your back straight and feet flat on the ground, hip-width apart.
- Engage your core to maintain an upright posture throughout the exercise.
- Place your hands on your thighs or the sides of the chair for added stability.

## EXECUTION

1. Extend your right leg out in front of you, keeping it slightly lifted off the floor.
2. Begin to draw circles in the air with your toes, initiating the movement from your hip to ensure full leg engagement.
3. Make 5-10 clockwise circles, keeping the movement smooth and controlled.
4. Pause briefly, then switch directions, making 5-10 counterclockwise circles with the same leg.
5. Lower your right leg back to the starting position and repeat the exercise with your left leg.
6. Aim to complete 2-3 sets for each leg.

# Chair Hip-Opening Side Stretch

**PURPOSE:** To improve flexibility, open the hips, and stretch the sides of the body while promoting relaxation and posture alignment.

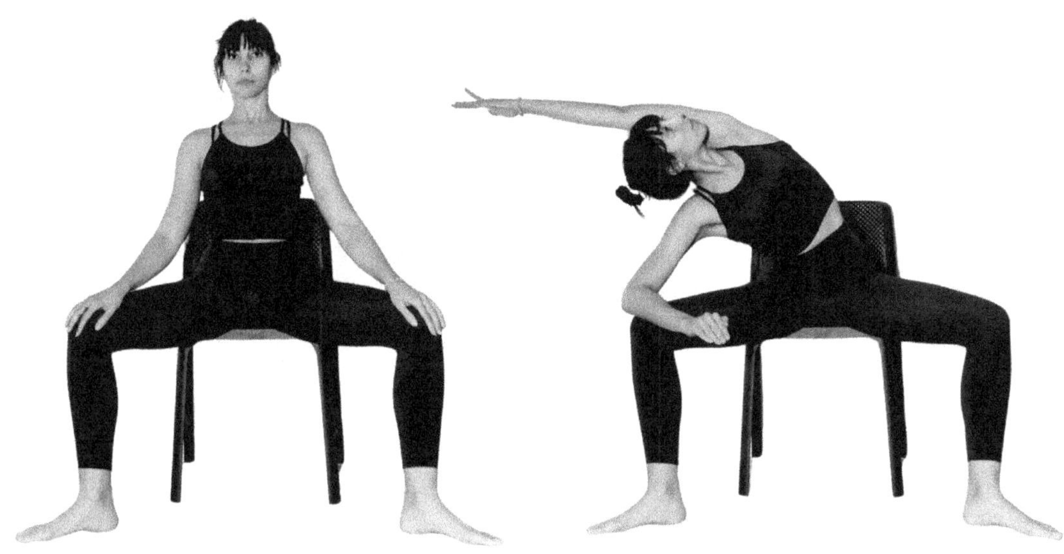

## PREPARATION

- Sit comfortably on a sturdy chair with your back straight and feet flat on the floor.
- Position yourself near the front edge of the chair to allow for greater mobility during the exercise.

## EXECUTION

1. Spread your legs wide, keeping feet firmly planted and knees aligned with toes. Rest your hands on your thighs, keeping your back straight and shoulders relaxed.
2. Breathe deeply.
3. Rest your right forearm on your right thigh and extend your left arm overhead, leaning gently to the right. Feel the stretch along the left side of your body. Hold for a few breaths, then repeat on the other side.

### Tips and Advice to Avoid Common Mistakes

Avoid overextending; stay within your comfort zone.

# Seated Warrior II Pose

**PURPOSE:** To improve hip flexibility, strengthen legs and arms, and enhance balance and focus through a dynamic seated warrior pose.

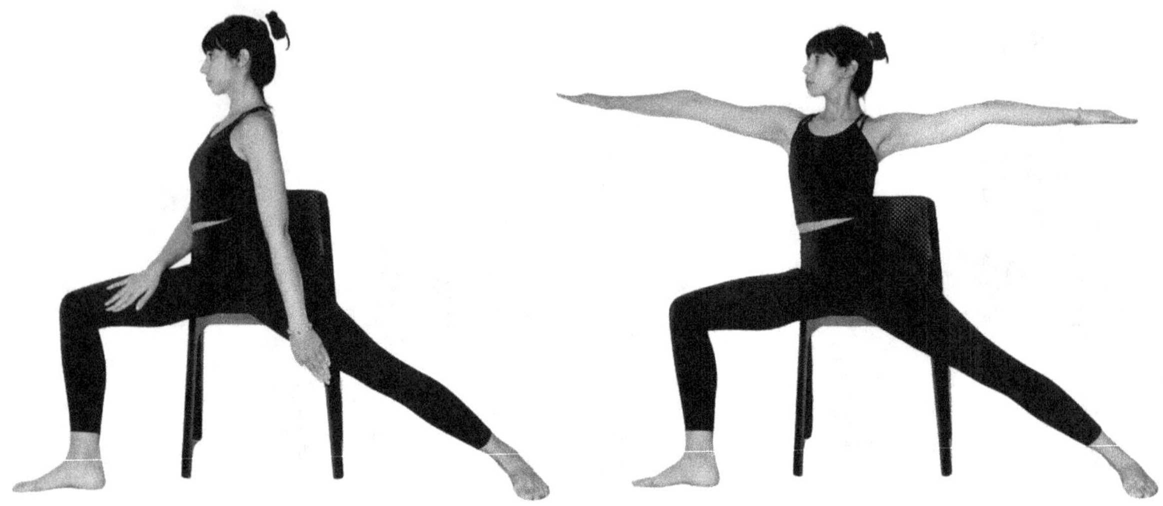

## PREPARATION

- Sit comfortably on a sturdy chair with your back straight and feet flat on the floor.
- Ensure you have enough space to extend one leg to the side during the exercise.

## EXECUTION

1. Sit upright with your legs slightly apart and your hands resting on your thighs. Breathe deeply to prepare.
2. Widen your stance by spreading your legs apart, keeping your feet firmly on the floor and knees aligned with your toes. Place your hands on your thighs for support and maintain a straight back.
3. Extend your right leg fully to the side, keeping your left knee bent at a 90-degree angle. Stretch your arms out to the sides, parallel to the floor, and gaze over your right hand. Feel the strength in your legs and the stretch in your hips. Hold for a few breaths, then switch sides.

# Seated Cross-Body Reach

**PURPOSE:** To engage and strengthen the core muscles, improve coordination, and enhance upper body mobility.

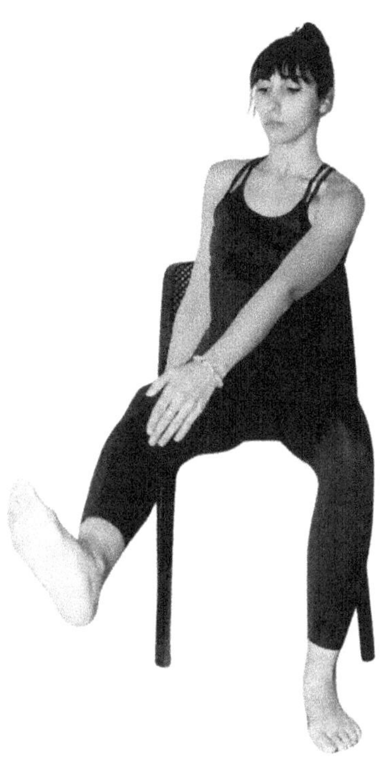 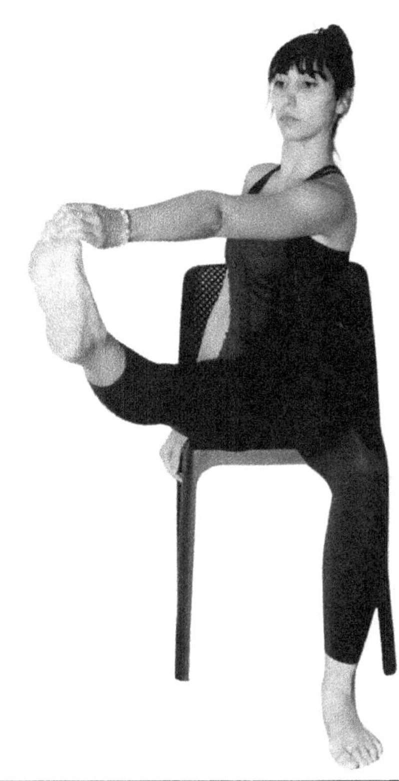

## PREPARATION

- Sit in a sturdy, armless chair with your feet flat on the ground, hip-width apart.
- Keep your back straight, engaging your core to support your upper body.
- Relax your shoulders down away from your ears, and place your hands on your lap.

## EXECUTION

1. Extend your right arm across your body towards the left side, while simultaneously lifting and extending your left leg straight out to the side.
2. Reach your right hand towards your left foot, creating a diagonal line across your body. If you cannot touch your foot, aim to reach in the direction of your toes.
3. Hold the reach for 2-3 seconds, focusing on stretching and engaging the muscles along your side and core.
4. Slowly return to the starting position and repeat the movement with your left arm and right leg.
5. Aim for 8-10 repetitions on each side, ensuring smooth and controlled movements throughout the exercise.

# Seated Leg and Arm Extension

**PURPOSE:** To engage and strengthen the core, improve coordination, and increase flexibility in the legs and arms.

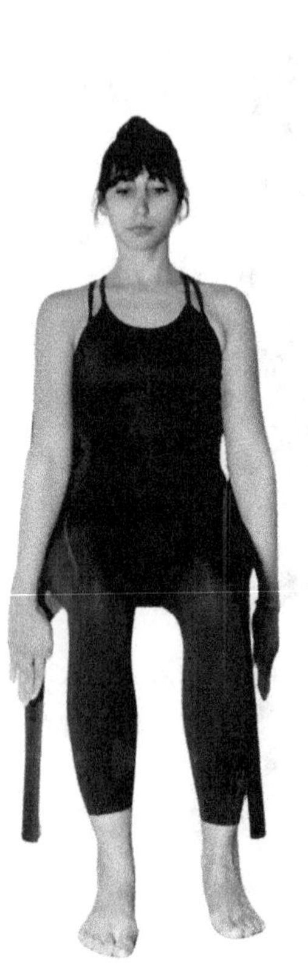 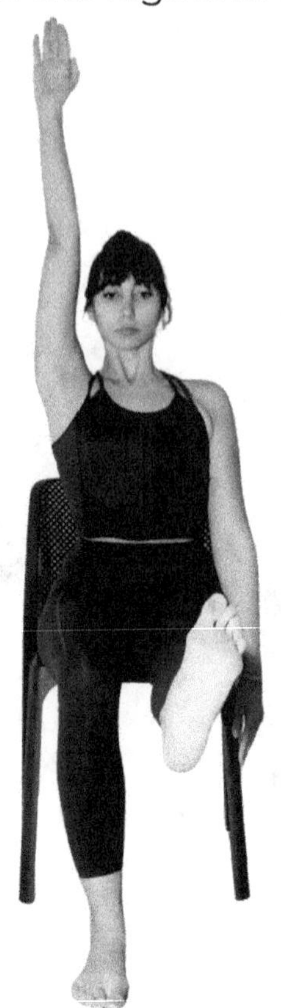

## PREPARATION

- Sit at the edge of a sturdy, armless chair with your feet flat on the ground, hip-width apart.
- Keep your back straight, engaging your core muscles to support your spine.
- Rest your hands on the sides of the chair for stability.

## EXECUTION

1. Extend your right arm upwards while simultaneously extending your left leg straight out in front of you, keeping your foot flexed.
2. Hold this position for 3-5 seconds, focusing on stretching both your arm and leg away from each other.
3. Slowly lower your arm and leg back to the starting position.
4. Repeat the movement with your left arm and right leg, ensuring smooth and controlled movements.
5. Aim for 10-15 repetitions on each side, alternating smoothly between sides.

# Seated Arm and Leg Pull

**PURPOSE:** To engage and strengthen the core, improve coordination, and enhance upper body strength.

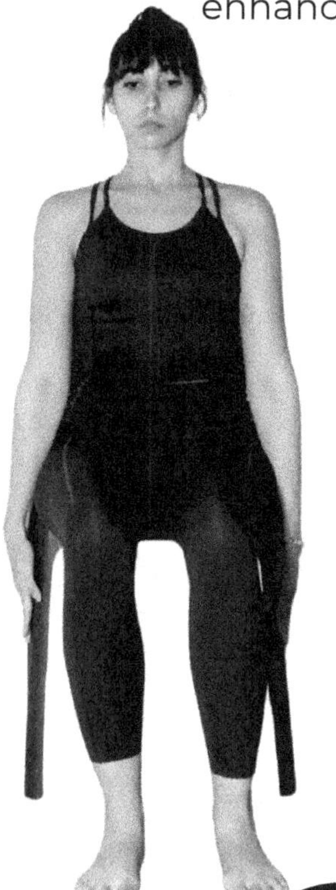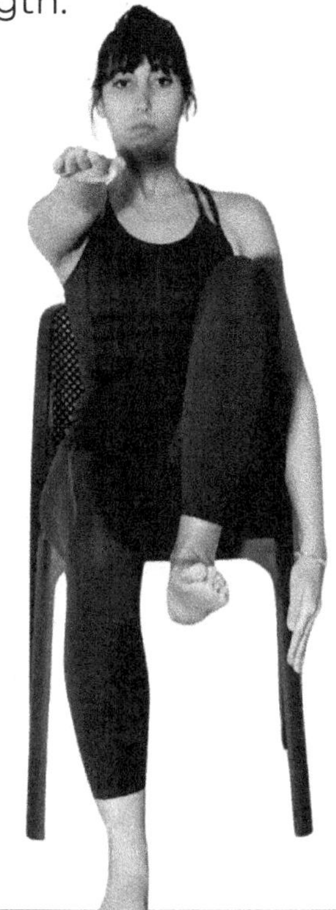

## PREPARATION

- Sit in a sturdy, armless chair at the edge, ensuring your feet can touch the floor comfortably.
- Keep your back straight, engaging your abdominal muscles slightly to maintain good posture.
- Rest your hands on the sides of the chair for initial balance.

## EXECUTION

1. Start by lifting your right arm and left leg simultaneously. Extend your right arm forward at shoulder height and lift your left knee towards the chest.
2. Hold the position for a count of two, focusing on the stretch and contraction in your muscles.
3. Slowly lower your right arm and left leg back to the starting position.
4. Repeat the movement with your left arm and right leg, lifting them simultaneously and holding for a count of two.
5. Continue alternating sides for 10-15 repetitions on each side, aiming for smooth and controlled movements throughout the exercise.
6. To maintain balance and coordination, focus on the opposite arm and leg moving together in a synchronized manner.

# Seated Full-Body Twist



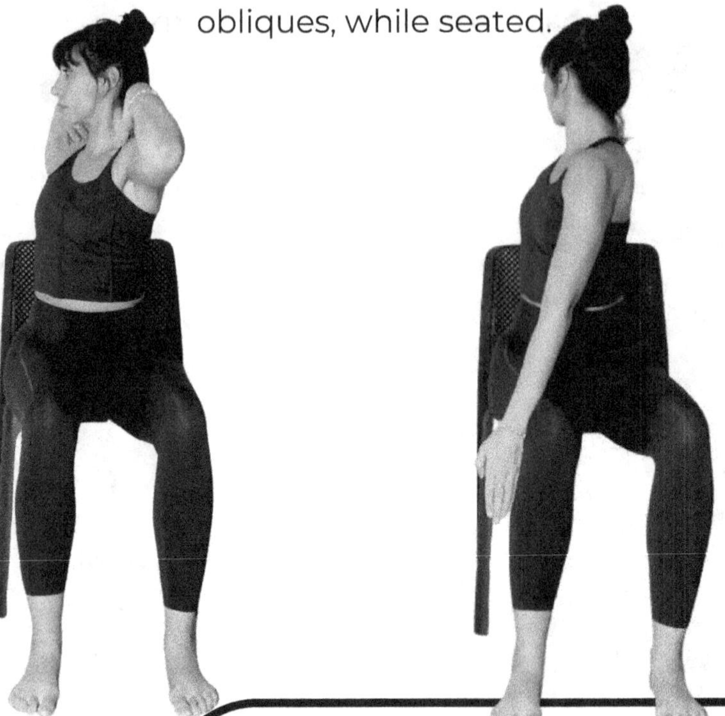

## PREPARATION

- Sit on the edge of a sturdy, armless chair with your feet planted firmly on the ground, hip-width apart.
- Keep your back straight, engaging your core muscles.
- Place your hands on your shoulders or extend your arms out to the sides at shoulder height, whichever feels more comfortable.

## EXECUTION

1. Inhale deeply, preparing your body for the twist.
2. As you exhale, gently twist your torso to the right, aiming to turn from your waist while keeping your hips and legs facing forward.
3. Extend your left hand towards your right knee, and if your arms are extended, follow the twist with your gaze, looking towards your right hand.
4. Hold this twisted position for 3-5 seconds, breathing deeply and focusing on the stretch along your spine and sides.
5. Inhale as you slowly return to the center, untwisting your torso.
6. Repeat the twist on the left side, this time extending your right hand towards your left knee and looking towards your left hand if your arms are extended.
7. Perform 5-10 repetitions on each side, ensuring smooth and controlled movements throughout the exercise.

# Seated Arm and Leg Balance

**PURPOSE:** To enhance coordination, balance, and strength throughout the body by engaging both the arms and legs simultaneously.

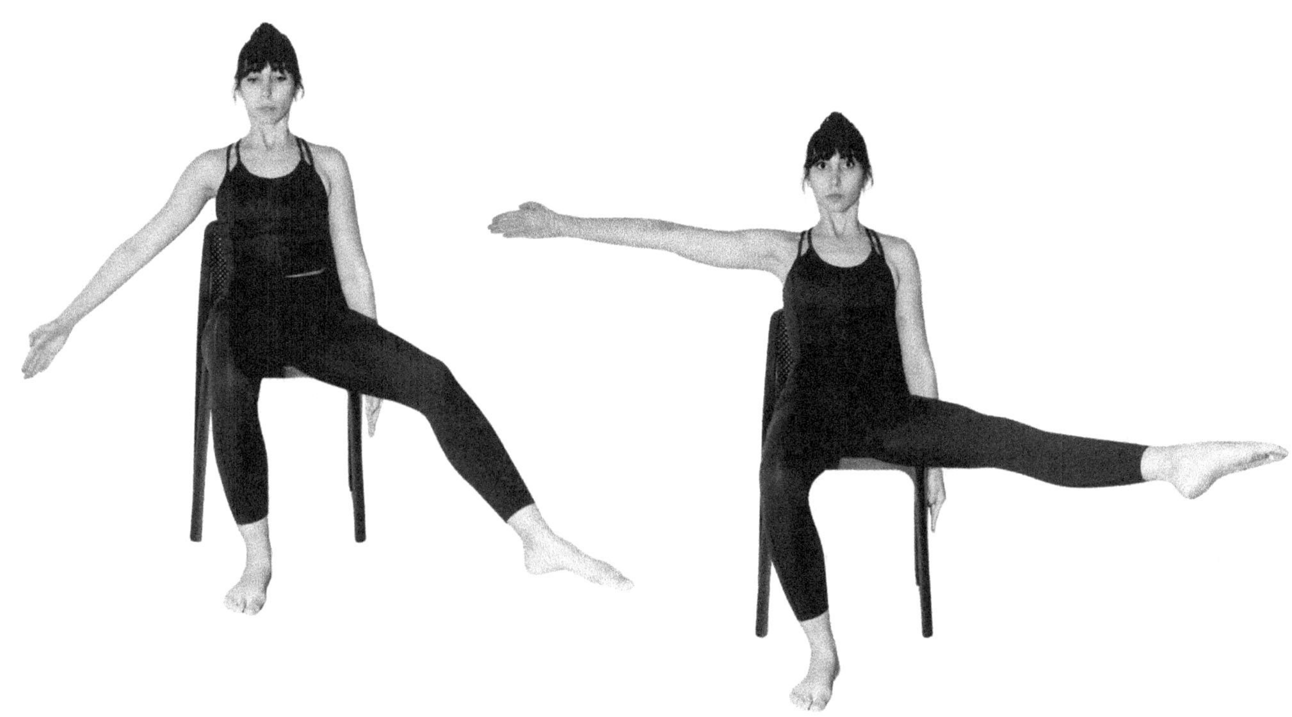

## PREPARATION

- Sit in a sturdy, armless chair with your feet flat on the ground, hip-width apart.
- Keep your back straight and engage your core to support your spine.
- Extend your arms alongside your body, palms facing down.

## EXECUTION

1. Slowly lift your right arm and left leg at the same time, extending them straight out to maintain balance.
2. Keep your arm and leg parallel to the floor, holding the position for a count of 3-5 seconds.
3. Carefully lower your arm and leg back to the starting position.
4. Repeat the movement with your left arm and right leg.
5. Aim for 5-10 repetitions on each side, focusing on maintaining a controlled and steady movement throughout the exercise.

# Seated Full-Body Flow

**PURPOSE:** To engage and activate the entire body in a gentle yet effective way, promoting weight loss, improving flexibility, and enhancing circulation, all from the safety and comfort of a chair.

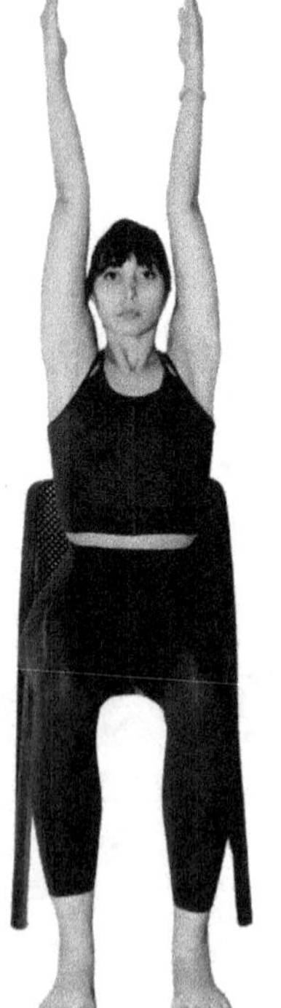 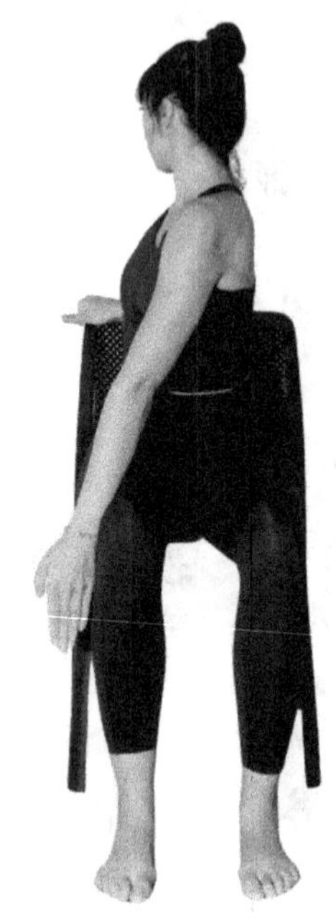

## PREPARATION

- Choose a stable chair without arms and sit at the edge with feet flat on the ground, hip-width apart.
- Sit up tall, engaging your core to support your spine.
- Relax your shoulders down away from your ears, and place your hands on your thighs.

## EXECUTION

1. Start by inhaling deeply and raising both arms overhead, stretching your spine and reaching towards the ceiling.
2. As you exhale, gently twist your torso to the right, lowering your arms to shoulder height, with your right hand reaching towards the back of the chair and your left hand towards your right knee.
3. Inhale as you return to the center, raising your arms overhead once again.
4. Exhale and repeat the twist to the left side, this time with your left hand reaching towards the back of the chair and your right hand towards your left knee.
5. After returning to the center with a deep inhale and arms raised, exhale and perform a forward bend, hinging at your hips and lowering your torso towards your thighs, allowing your arms to dangle towards the floor.
6. Inhale, slowly rolling up to a seated position, and finish by stretching both arms overhead once more.
7. Repeat the entire sequence 3-5 times, moving fluidly from one movement to the next, creating a flow.

# Relaxation and Recovery

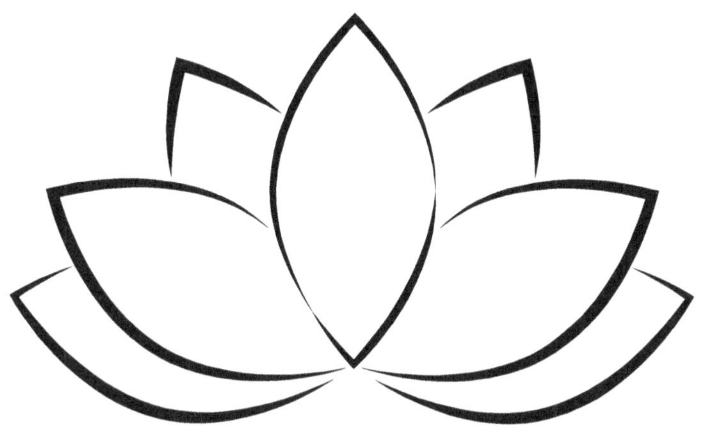

Scan the QR code to view the 5 exercises included in this section.

# Seated Relaxation Pose

**PURPOSE:** To promote relaxation and recovery, reducing stress and tension in the body.

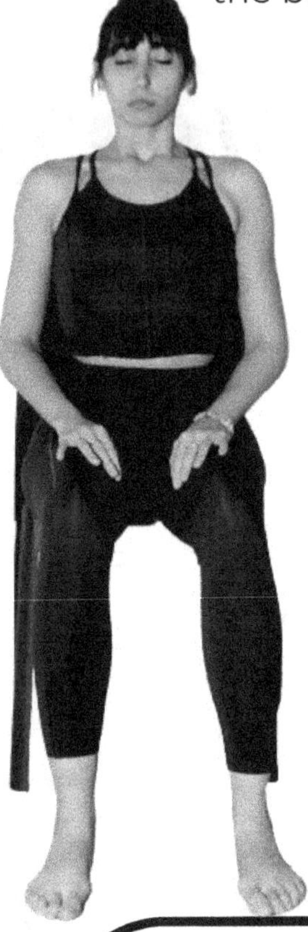

## PREPARATION

- Choose a comfortable, sturdy chair positioned in a quiet, distraction-free area.
- Sit in the chair with your feet flat on the floor, hip-width apart, and hands resting gently on your thighs.
- Straighten your spine, roll your shoulders back and down, and gently close your eyes to begin focusing inward.

## EXECUTION

1. Take a deep breath in, filling your lungs fully and expanding your chest.
2. As you exhale, consciously relax your shoulders, letting go of any tension held in your neck and upper back.
3. Continue to breathe deeply and evenly, focusing on the sensation of air moving in and out of your body. With each exhale, allow yourself to sink deeper into a state of relaxation.
4. If your mind begins to wander, gently redirect your focus back to your breath, using it as an anchor to the present moment.
5. Remain in this relaxed state for 5-10 minutes, allowing the calmness to permeate through your body.

# Seated Shoulder Stretch

**PURPOSE:** To improve shoulder mobility, stretch the upper body, and enhance posture while promoting relaxation.

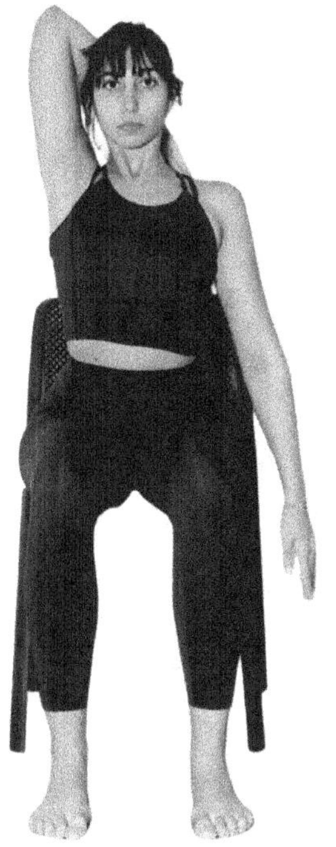 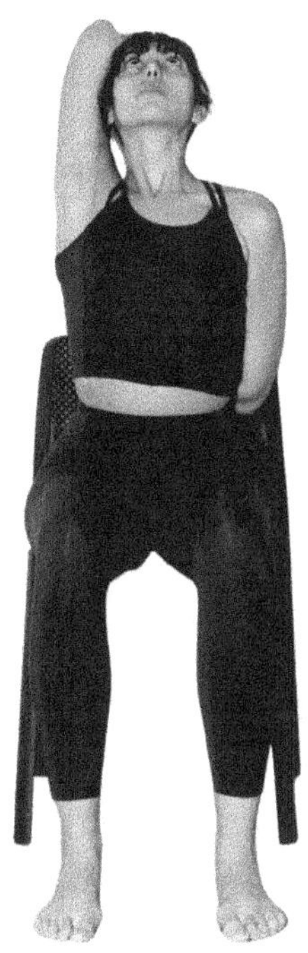

## PREPARATION

- Sit comfortably on a sturdy chair with your back straight and feet flat on the floor.
- Relax your shoulders and let your arms hang naturally at your sides.

## EXECUTION

1. Sit tall with your arms resting naturally at your sides. Take a deep breath to center yourself.
2. Raise your right arm upward toward the ceiling, keeping it straight, and let your left arm remain by your side. Hold for a moment and breathe deeply.
3. Bend your right elbow and place your hand behind your head. Extend your left arm outward to the side, creating a stretch through the shoulders and upper body.
4. Reach your right hand further down behind your back while bending your left arm behind your waist to meet your right hand. If possible, clasp your hands together or simply reach as close as you can. Breathe deeply and hold.
5. Release your hands and return to the starting position. Repeat the same sequence on the opposite side.

# Seated Calming Breath

**PURPOSE:** To calm the mind and body, reduce stress, and improve oxygen flow throughout the body, aiding in relaxation and recovery after a series of more active exercises.

## PREPARATION
- Sit comfortably in a sturdy chair without arms, ensuring your feet are flat on the ground, hip-width apart.
- Rest your hands on your lap, palms facing up or down based on personal comfort.
- Straighten your spine but avoid stiffening your back; maintain a relaxed but upright posture.
- Close your eyes gently to minimize external distractions and focus inward.

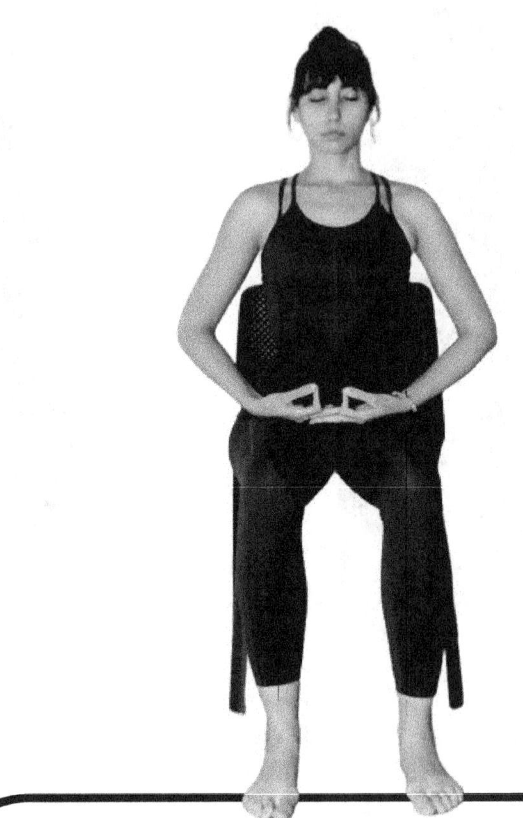

## EXECUTION
1. Begin by taking a deep breath in through your nose, allowing your chest and belly to expand fully.
2. Hold the breath for a count of three.
3. Exhale slowly through your mouth, focusing on releasing all the air from your lungs and feeling the relaxation spreading through your body.
4. After fully exhaling, pause for a moment before taking another breath.
5. Continue this breathing pattern for 3-5 minutes, concentrating on the sensation of each breath filling and leaving your body.
6. If your mind wanders, gently redirect your focus back to your breath, using it as an anchor to the present moment.

# Seated Mindful Stretch

**PURPOSE:** To gently stretch and relax the entire body, focusing on releasing tension and promoting a sense of calm. This exercise is designed to enhance mindfulness and body awareness, contributing to stress reduction and overall well-being.

## PREPARATION

- Sit comfortably in a sturdy, armless chair with your feet flat on the ground, hip-width apart.
- Keep your back straight but not stiff, and place your hands on your thighs or knees, palms down.
- Close your eyes gently to enhance focus on bodily sensations and breathing.

## EXECUTION

1. Take a deep breath in, filling your lungs completely, and hold for a count of three.
2. As you exhale slowly, focus on releasing tension in your shoulders, neck, and back. Imagine the stress leaving your body with each breath out.
3. Continue to breathe deeply and at a steady pace, directing your attention to different parts of your body. With each exhale, visualize tension melting away from each area you focus on.
4. After several breaths, shift your focus to your seated posture. Feel the chair supporting your weight and the ground beneath your feet.
5. Maintain this mindful state, breathing deeply and evenly, for 5-10 minutes. With each breath, aim to deepen your sense of relaxation and presence.

# Seated Relaxation Flow

**PURPOSE:** To gently relax the body and mind.

**PREPARATION:** Sit tall, feet flat, hands on lap, breathe deeply.

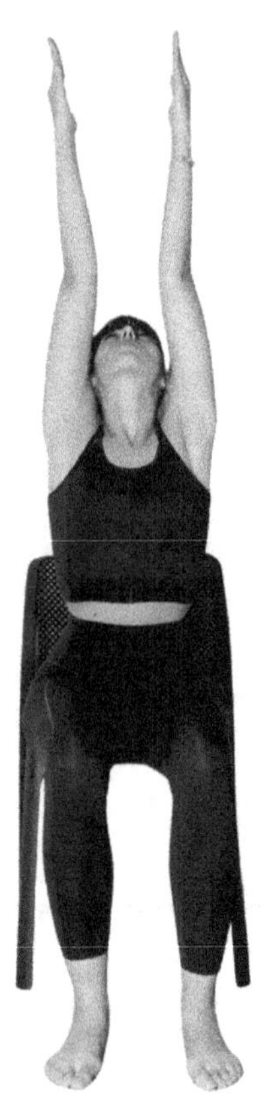

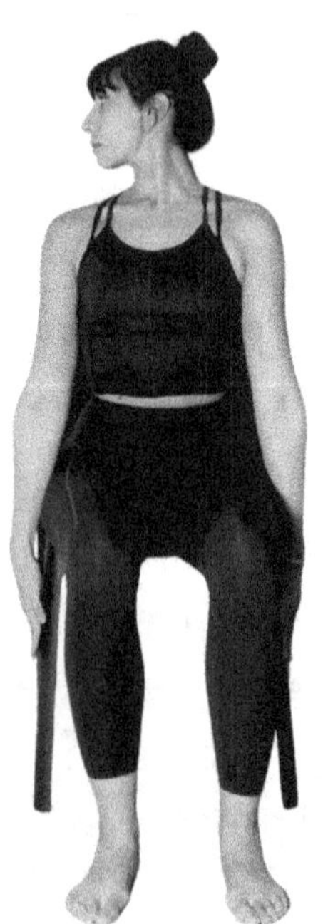

### EXECUTION

1. Inhale deeply, raising both arms overhead, palms facing each other, stretching the spine and opening the chest.
2. Exhale slowly, lowering your arms back to your lap, focusing on the sensation of release throughout your body.
3. Inhale, gently turn your head to the right, aiming for a comfortable stretch in your neck.
4. Exhale, return your head to the center.
5. Inhale, turn your head to the left, maintaining a smooth, gentle motion.
6. Exhale, bring your head back to the center.
7. Inhale, extend your right leg out in front of you, foot flexed, engaging the leg muscles.
8. Exhale, slowly lower your right leg back to the starting position.
9. Inhale, repeat the leg extension with your left leg, focusing on the stretch and engagement.
10. Exhale, return your left leg to the starting position.
11. Inhale deeply, and as you exhale, gently lean forward from your hips, reaching toward your toes, keeping your back straight.
12. Hold this forward bend for a few breaths, allowing your body to relax into the stretch.
13. Inhale, slowly rise back to a seated position, raising your arms overhead once more.
14. Exhale, lower your arms and gently close your eyes, taking a few moments to breathe deeply and relax fully.

# Chapter 5: Quick Workouts for Busy Days

For those days when time is of the essence, but the commitment to health and weight loss remains a priority, a series of 10-minute chair yoga sessions can be a game-changer. These quick workouts are designed to fit seamlessly into your busy schedule, ensuring that you can maintain consistency in your exercise routine without the need for extensive preparation or recovery time. The beauty of chair yoga lies in its accessibility and adaptability, making it an ideal choice for seniors and beginners who are looking to embark on a weight loss journey without the risk of strain or injury.

The first routine we'll explore focuses on activating the body in the morning. This AM Routine is crafted to gently wake up the body, boost metabolism, and set a positive tone for the day ahead. It begins with a series of seated deep diaphragmatic breathing exercises to oxygenate the blood and awaken the senses. Following this, a sequence of gentle seated stretches such as the Seated Mountain Pose and Seated Cat-Cow Stretch helps to loosen any stiffness accumulated during sleep. Incorporating movements that target the core, such as the Seated Core Twist, not only engages the muscles but also stimulates digestion, which is crucial for weight management. Each exercise should be performed for approximately one minute, ensuring that you're fully present and mindful of your body's responses to each movement.

Transitioning to the PM Routine, the focus shifts towards unwinding and releasing the tensions of the day. This evening sequence includes exercises like the Seated Gentle Twist and Seated Forward Bend, which are excellent for relieving stress and calming the nervous system. The inclusion of the Seated Leg Lifts and Seated Arm Circles aids in maintaining muscle tone and flexibility, crucial components of a successful weight loss strategy. As with the morning routine, dedicating about one minute to each exercise allows for a balanced session that respects the body's need to relax and rejuvenate.

It's important to remember that the goal of these 10-minute sessions is not only to aid in weight loss but also to foster a deeper connection with the body. By integrating these short routines into your daily life, you're taking a step towards a more active, healthy, and balanced lifestyle. The simplicity and efficiency of chair yoga make it an empowering tool for those looking to lose weight, improve flexibility, and enhance overall well-being without the need for high-impact activities.

For those looking to elevate their fitness routine beyond the basics, incorporating Total Body Activation sessions can significantly enhance the chair yoga experience. The Low-Intensity Total Body Activation is meticulously designed to engage every major muscle group without overwhelming the body. Starting with Seated Side Leg Lifts and progressing through Seated Arm Raises, this routine emphasizes controlled movements to build strength and flexibility across the body. The inclusion of Seated Knee Tucks will target the core, while Seated Ankle Circles ensure that even the often-neglected areas receive attention. Performing each exercise for around one minute encourages a thorough activation of the muscles, preparing them for more dynamic movements throughout the day.

Transitioning into the High-Intensity Total Body Activation, the pace and complexity of the exercises increase slightly to challenge the body further. This segment introduces Seated Bicycle Crunches and Seated Leg Extensions, pushing the boundaries of what can be achieved within the confines of a chair. The Seated Full-Body Stretch and Seated Arm and Leg Reach are integrated to ensure that flexibility is maintained even as the intensity escalates. This high-energy routine is perfect for those days when you're seeking a more vigorous session, aiming to maximize calorie burn and muscle engagement within the same ten-minute framework.

Muscle Toning sessions are another critical component of a comprehensive chair yoga routine, with both Low and High-Intensity options available. The Low-Intensity Muscle Toning focuses on gentle, sustained movements like the Seated Inner Thigh Squeeze and Seated Glute Squeeze, which are fantastic for sculpting muscles without strain. On the other hand, the High-Intensity Muscle Toning incorporates Seated Russian Twists and Seated Leg and Arm Extension, ramping up the effort required and promising a more pronounced impact on muscle tone and definition.

For those days when the primary goal is to ignite the body's fat-burning capabilities, the Fat Burning Flow routines come into play. The Low-Intensity Fat Burning Flow is a carefully curated sequence that combines moderate aerobic exercises with strength training elements, ensuring a balanced approach to weight loss. The High-Intensity Fat Burning Flow, however, adopts a more aggressive strategy, integrating faster-paced movements and shorter rest periods to elevate the heart rate and stimulate a higher caloric burn.

Lastly, the Full Body Stretch routine is an essential element of any chair yoga regimen, designed to enhance mobility and reduce the risk of injury. This routine encompasses a variety of stretches that target the entire body, from the neck down to the toes, ensuring that each muscle group is properly elongated and relaxed. It serves as a perfect conclusion to any of the aforementioned routines or as a standalone session for days dedicated to recovery and flexibility.

By integrating these diverse routines into your weekly schedule, you can enjoy a holistic approach to fitness that addresses strength, flexibility, balance, and cardiovascular health. Chair yoga's versatility makes it an invaluable tool for seniors and beginners alike, offering a pathway to improved physical health and a more active lifestyle without the intimidation of traditional exercise regimens.

# WORKOUT 1 - AM ROUTINE

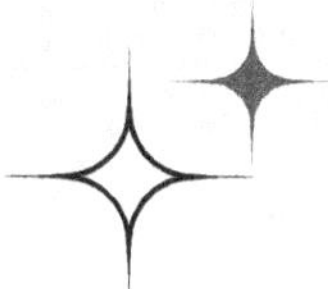

**Seated Mountain Pose**
Page 27

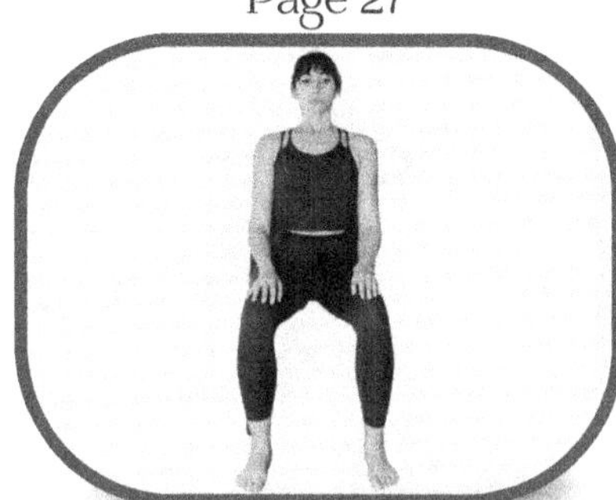

1 minute

**Seated Arm Circles**
Page 33

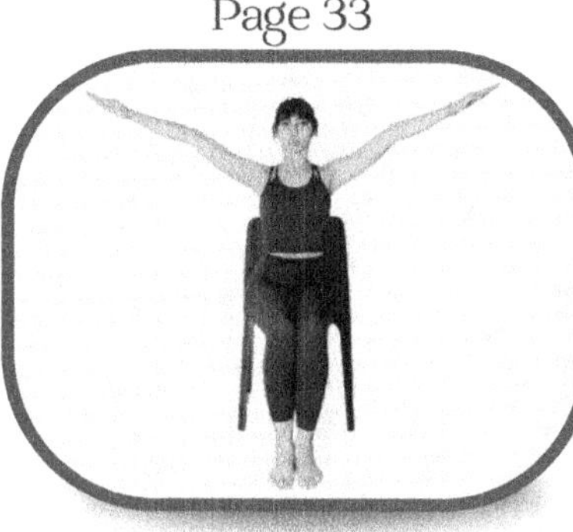

1 minute

**Seated Cat–Cow Stretch**
Page 28

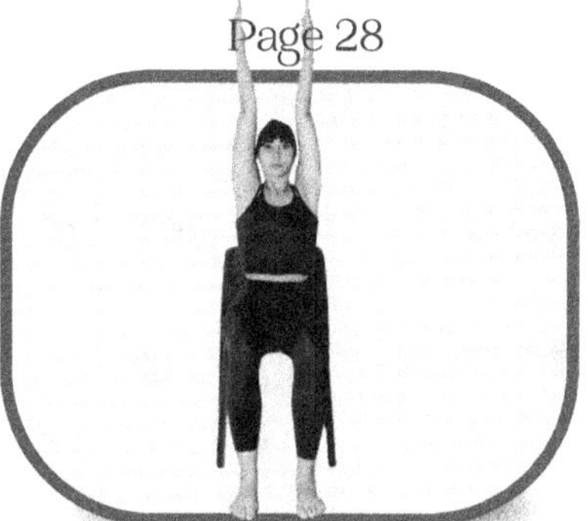

10 repetitions

**Seated Forward Bend**
Page 29

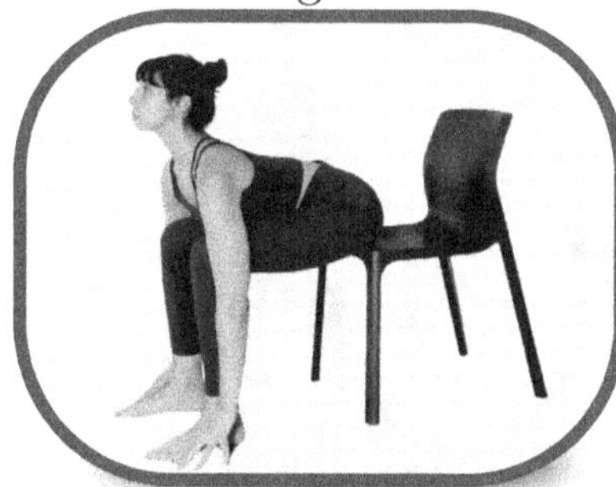

10 repetitions

**Seated Spinal Twist**
Page 30

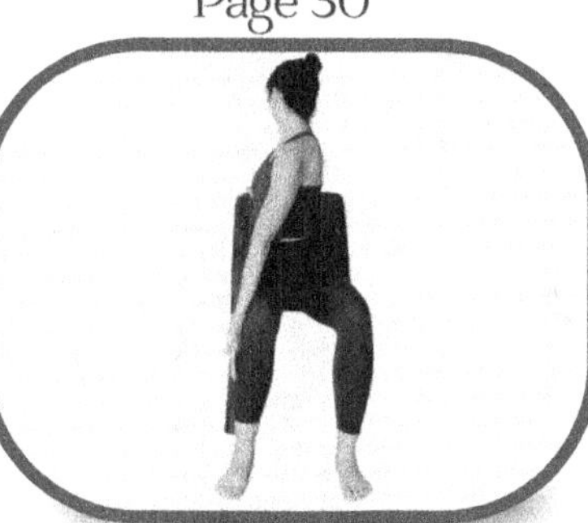

10 repetitions

**Seated Calming Breath**
Page 84

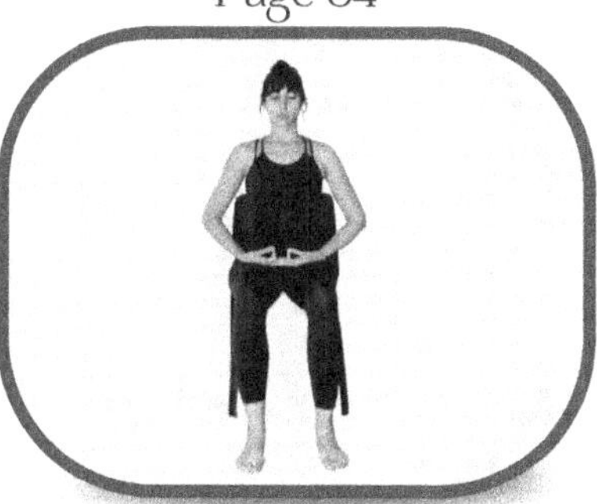

1 minute

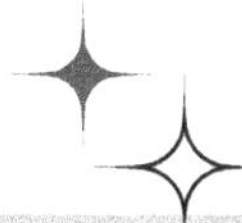

This routine is designed to gently activate the body, enhance flexibility, and kickstart the metabolism in a manner that is both effective and considerate of the physical limitations often present in seniors and beginners.

# WORKOUT 2 - PM ROUTINE

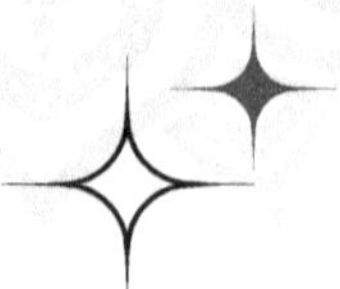

Seated Marching
Page 34

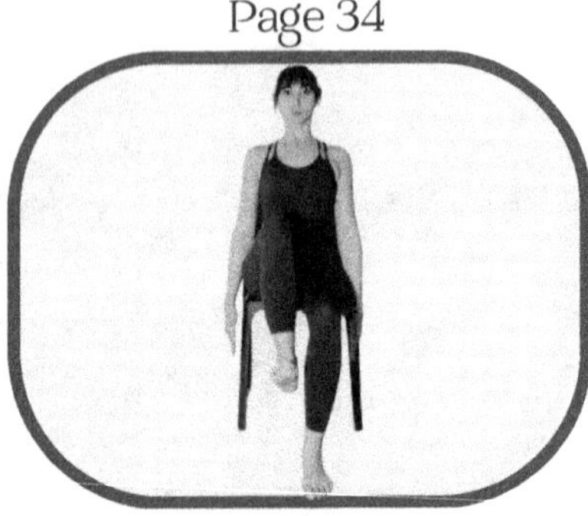

| 10 repetitions |

Seated Side Bend
Page 31

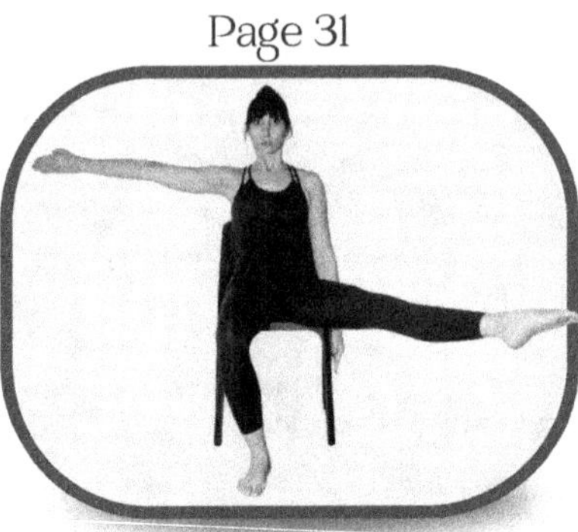

| 10 repetitions |

Seated Forward Bend
Page 29

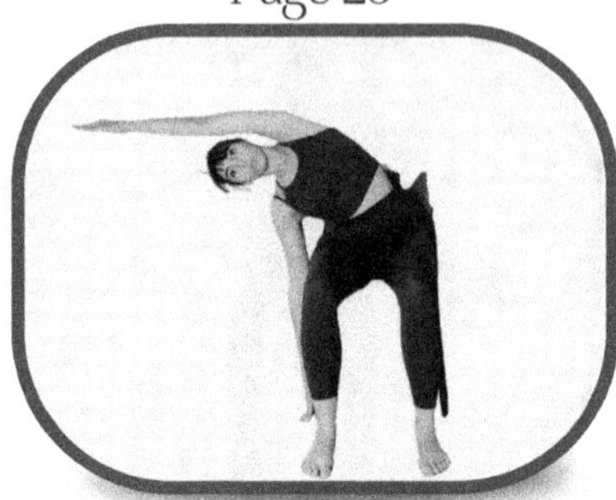

| 10 repetitions |

Seated Inner Thigh Squeeze
Page 64

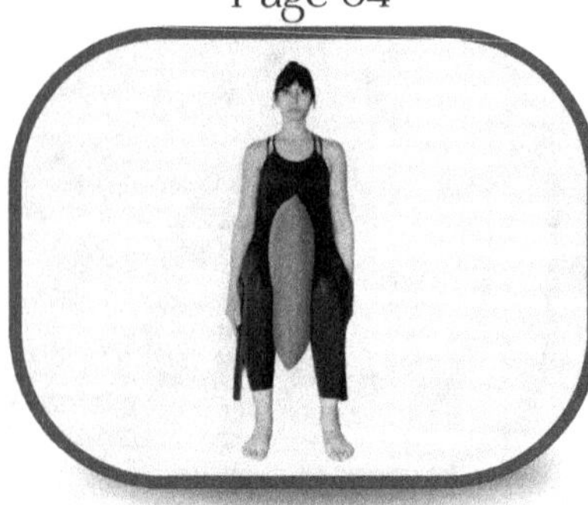

| 10 repetitions |

Seated Bicycle Crunches
Page 38

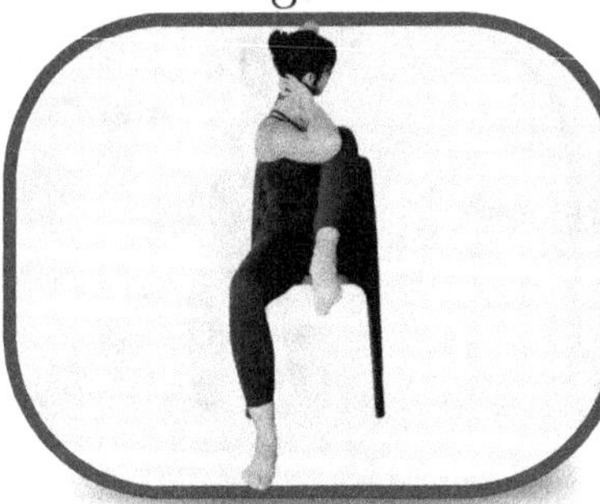

| 10 repetitions |

Seated Mindful Stretch
Page 85

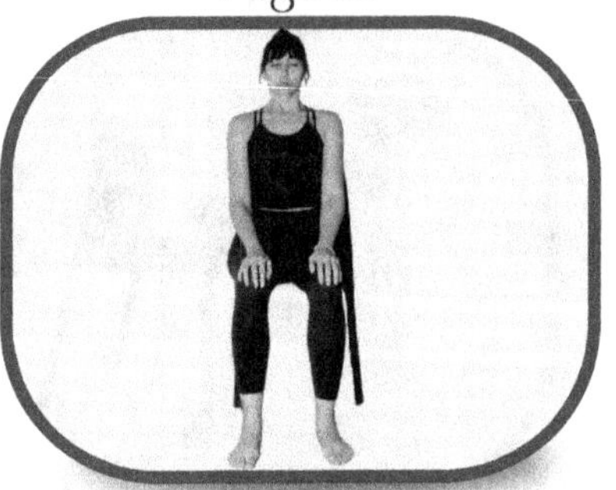

| 2 minutes |

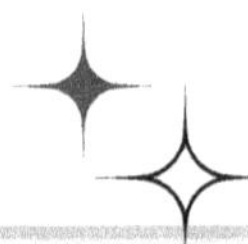

Continuing with the PM Routine, designed to help unwind and relax after a day's activities, this sequence focuses on releasing tension, improving flexibility, and maintaining muscle tone.

# WORKOUT 3
# TOTAL BODY ACTIVATION

Seated Marching
Page 34

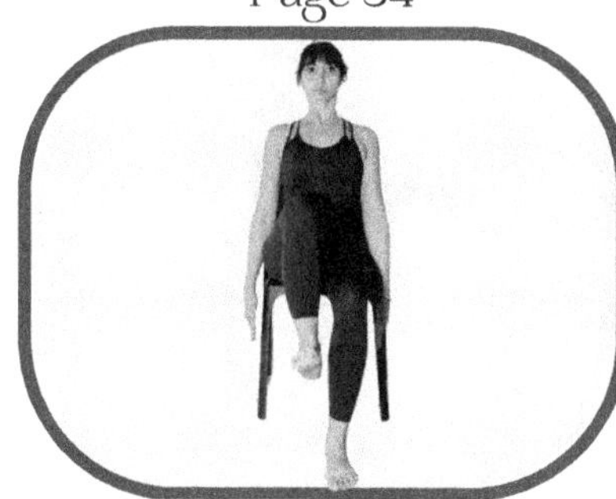

10 repetitions

Seated Bicycle Crunches:
Page 38

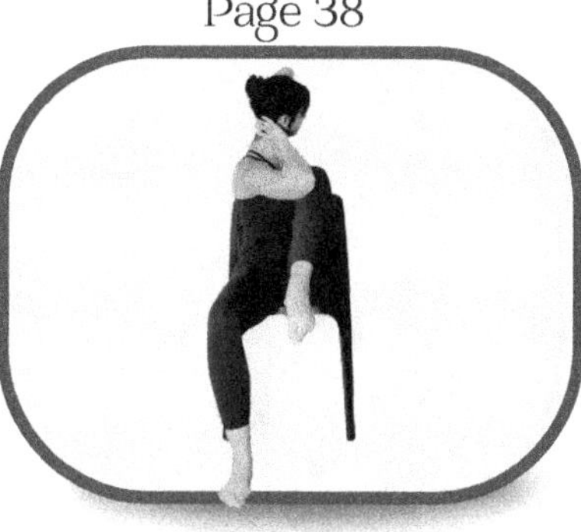

10 repetitions

Seated Leg Lifts
Page 32

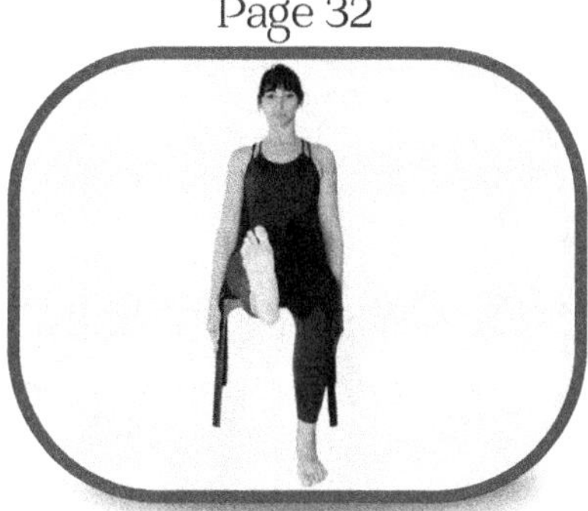

10 repetitions

Seated Russian Twists
Page 41

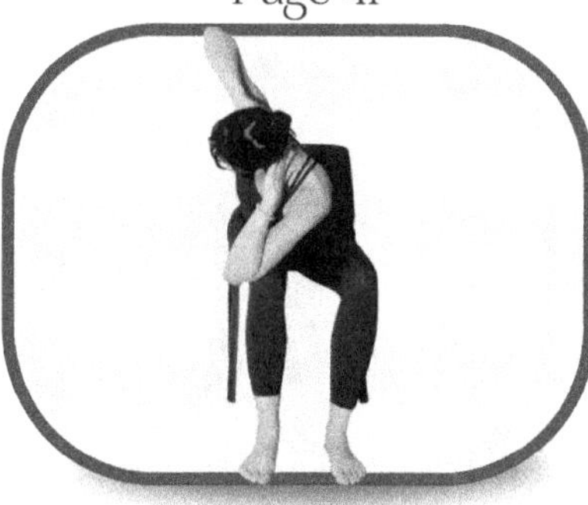

10 repetitions

Seated Knee Tucks
Page 40

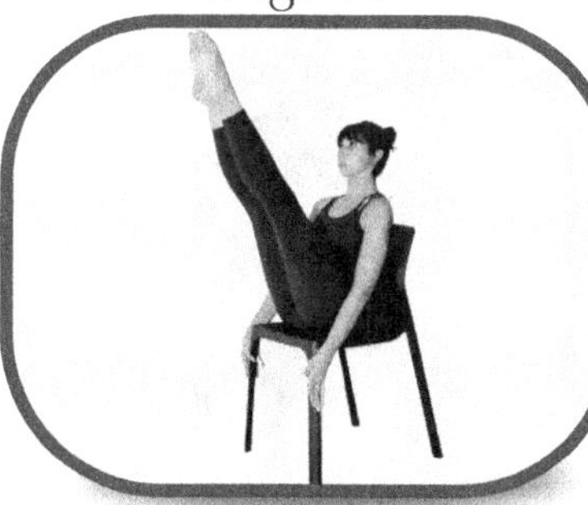

10 repetitions

Seated Full–Body Stretch
Page 69

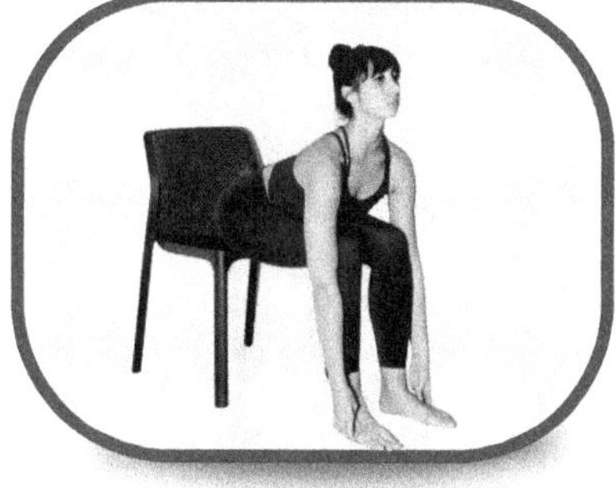

5 repetitions

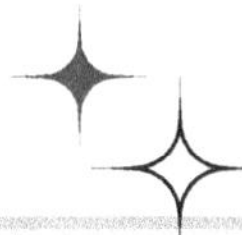

This routine builds on the foundational movements introduced in Chapter 4, emphasizing slow, controlled motions that target key muscle groups without overexertion. The goal is to enhance muscle tone, improve strength, and promote overall well–being.

# WORKOUT 4
# MUSCLE TONING ROUTINE

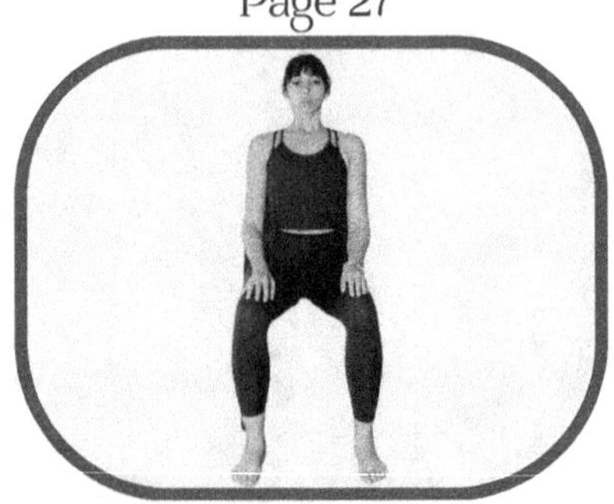

Seated Mountain Pose
Page 27

8 to 10 deep breaths

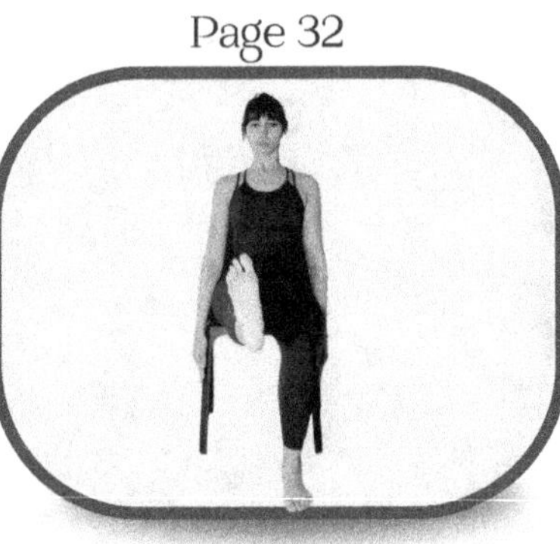

Seated Leg Lifts
Page 32

10 repetitions

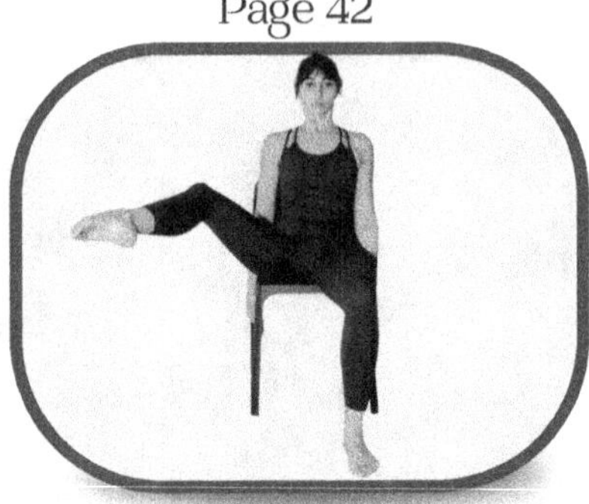

Seated Side Leg Lifts
Page 42

10 repetitions

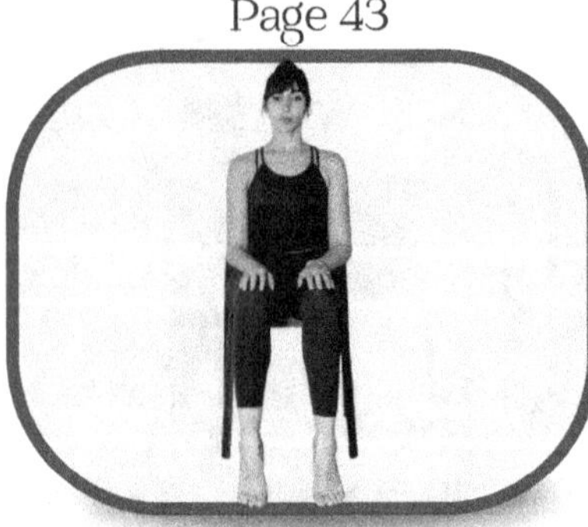

Seated Heel Raises
Page 43

5 repetitions

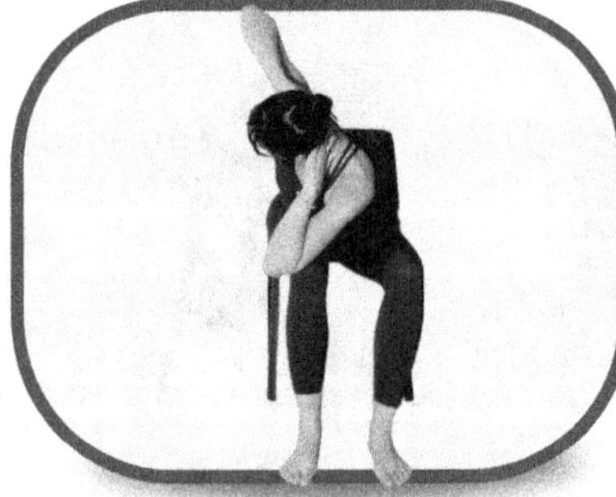

Seated Russian Twists
Page 41

10 repetitions

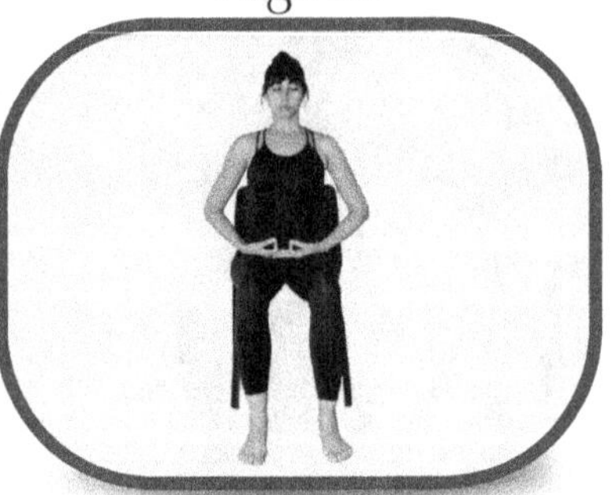

Seated Calming Breath
Page 84

2 minutes

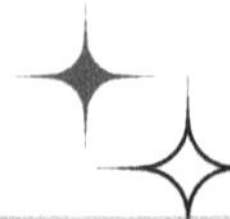

For the Full Body Stretch routine, it's crucial to focus on exercises that encompass the entire body, promoting flexibility, circulation, and relaxation. This routine is tailored specifically for those days when your body craves a gentle but thorough stretch,

# WORKOUT 5
# FAT BURNING FLOW ROUTINE

Seated Full-Body Flow
Page 80

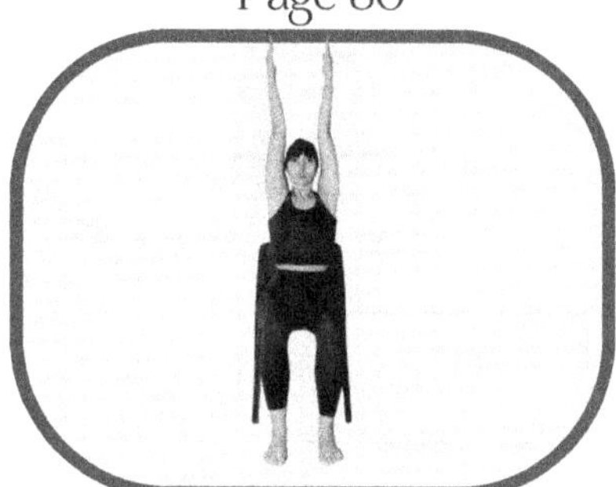

10 rotations

Seated Leg Circles
Page 72

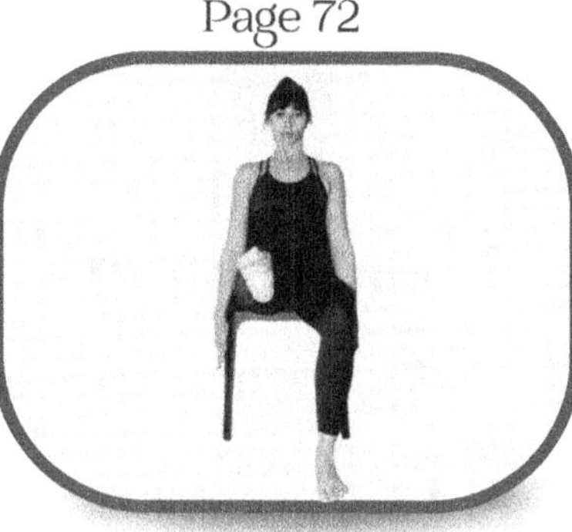

10 seconds clockwise, 10 seconds counterclockwise on each leg

Seated Full-Body Stretch
Page 69

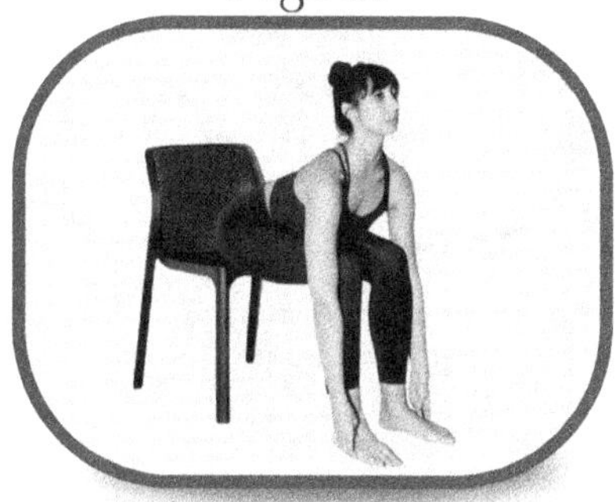

5 repetitions

Seated Leg and Arm
Extension - Page 76

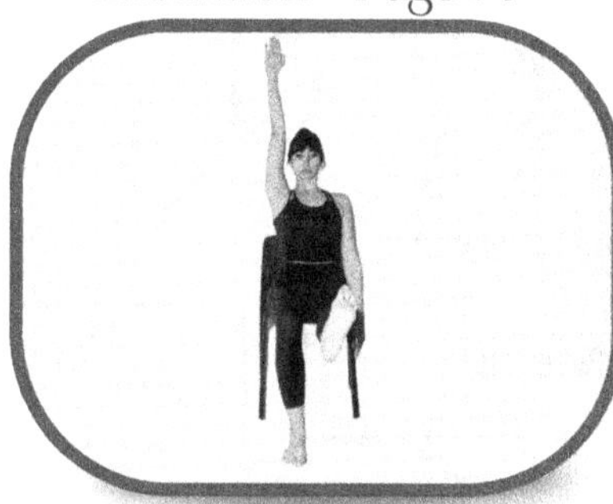

10 repetitions

Seated Cross-Body Reach
Page 75

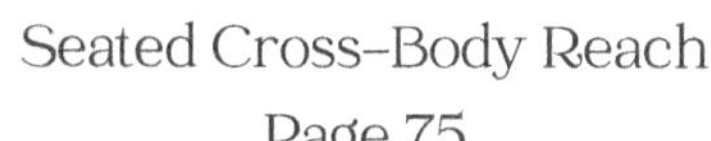
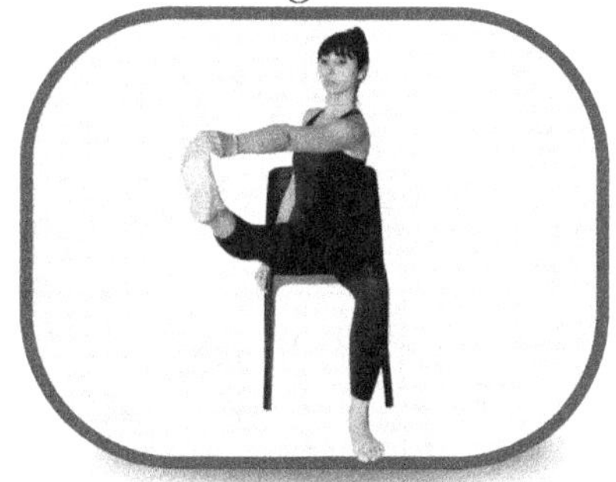

10 repetitions

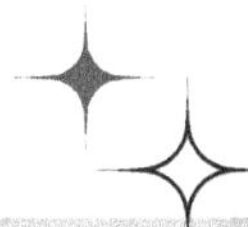

For the Fat Burning Flow Low Intensity routine, let's focus on a series of exercises that gently increase your heart rate, promote weight loss, and improve mobility without overexerting yourself.

# 6 - FULL BODY STRETCH ROUTINE

Seated Hip Flexor Stretch
Page 62

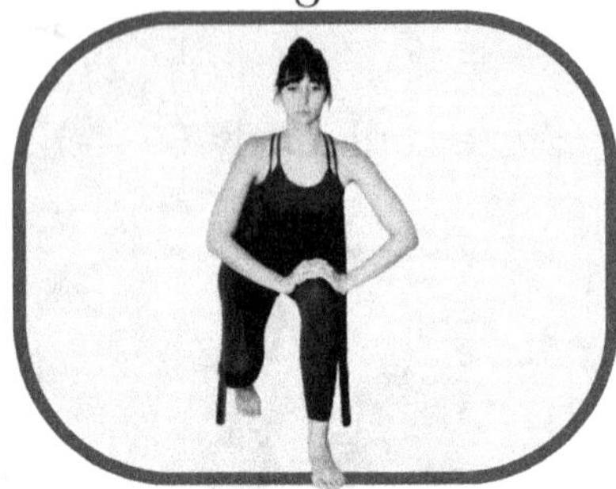

5 repetitions

Seated Leg and Arm
Extension – Page 76

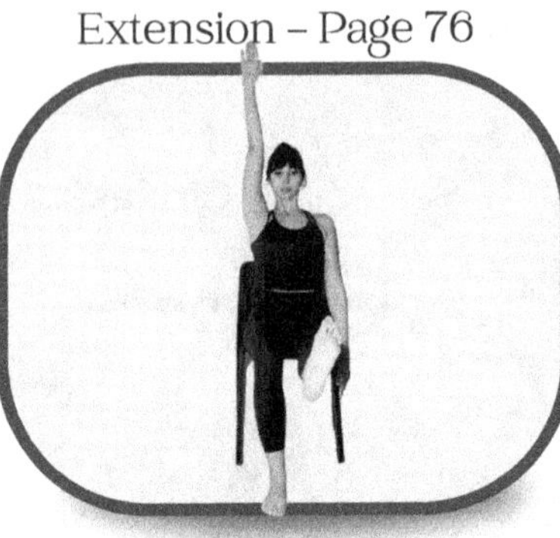

10 repetitions

Seated Full–Body Flow
Page 80

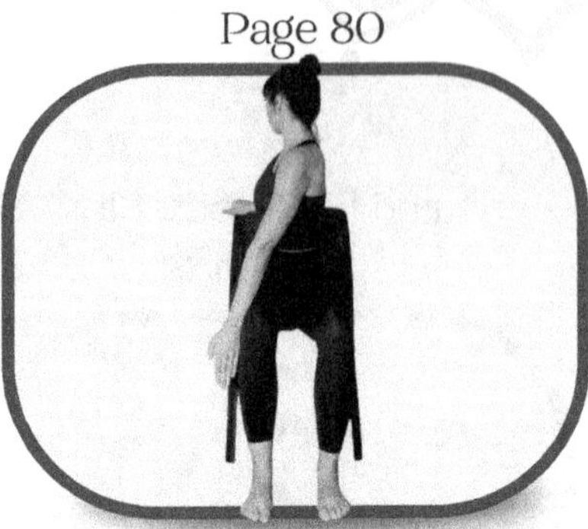

10 repetitions

Seated Leg Circles
Page 72

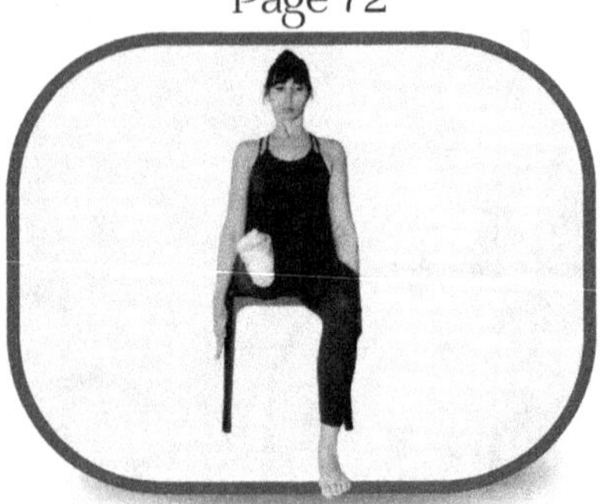

10 seconds clockwise, 10
seconds counterclockwise
on each leg

Seated Cross–Body Reach
Page 75

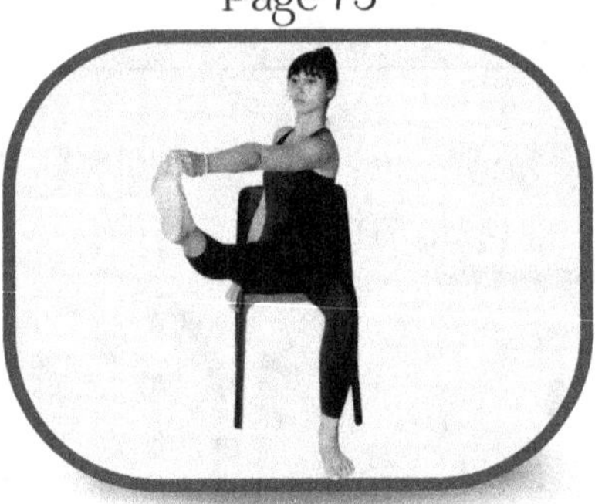

10 repetitions

Seated Arm and Leg Pull
Page 77

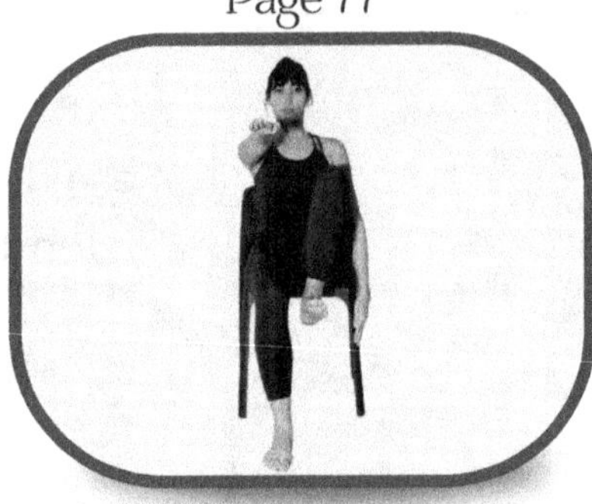

10 repetitions

Seated Relaxation Pose
Page 82

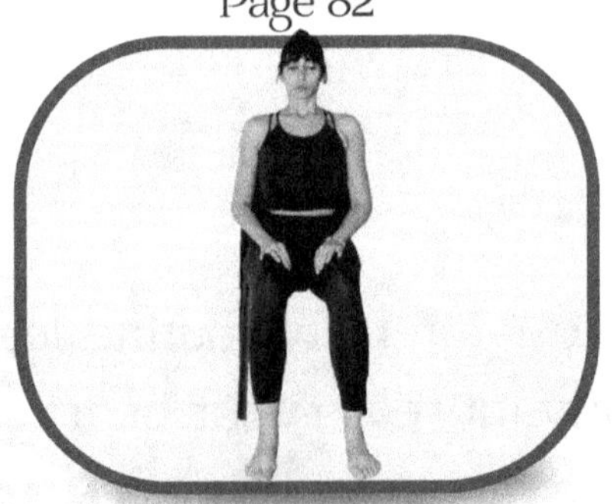

5 deep breaths

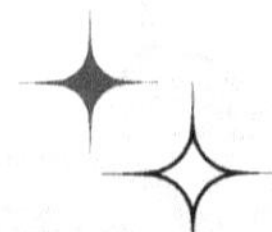

# 7 - ALL-IN-ONE YOGA PRACTICE

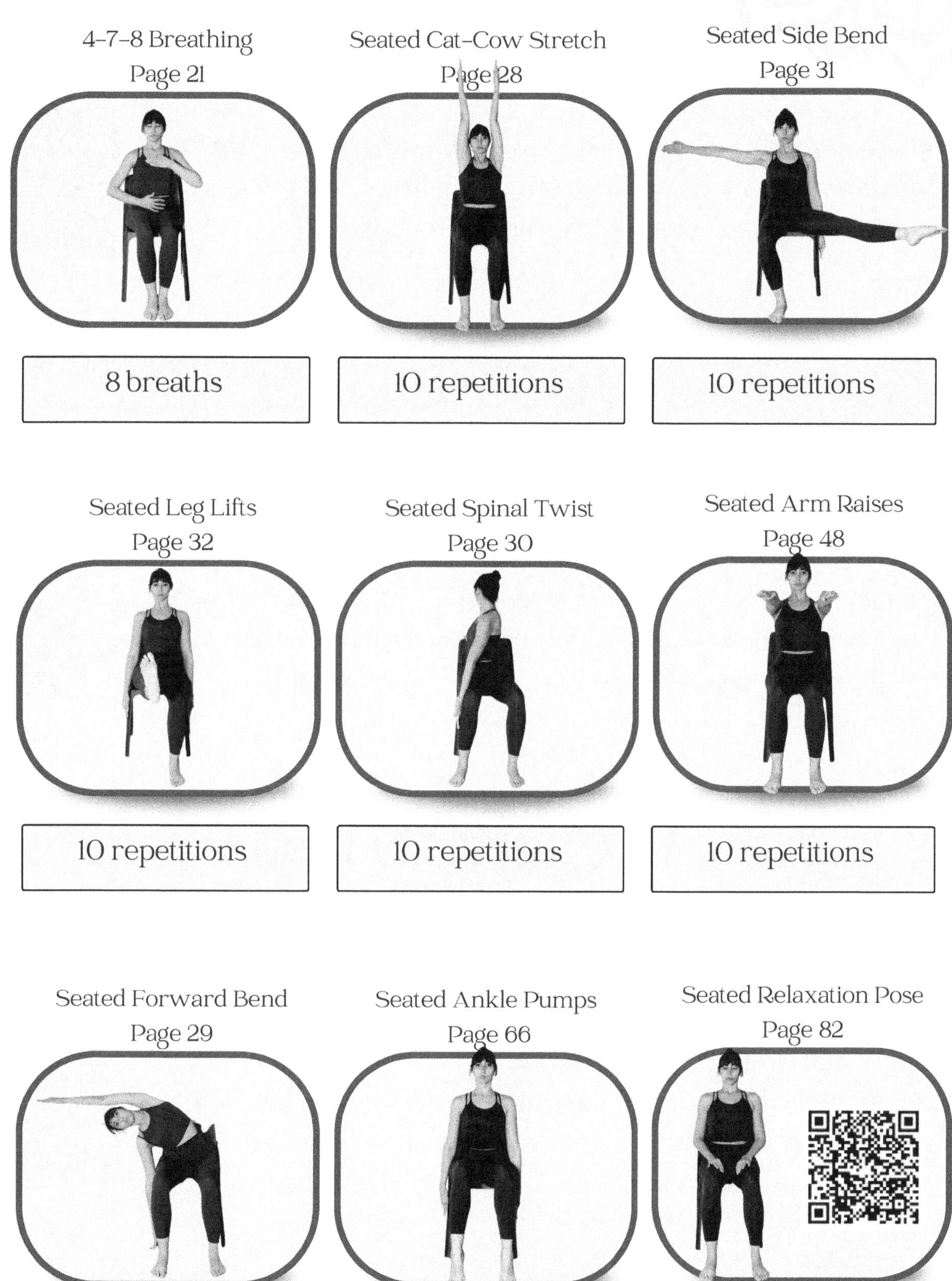

# WORKOUT 8
# RELAXATION ROUTINE

Whether you're looking to unwind after a long day or ease into a fitness journey, this routine offers a calming and effective solution for overall well-being.

# WORKOUT 9
# STANDING ROUTINE

This standing chair yoga sequence is ideal for enhancing balance, flexibility, and core strength. Using the chair as a support, the poses focus on controlled stretches and gentle movements, promoting stability and relaxation

# WORKOUT 10
# FULL-BODY CHAIR STRETCH

This seated routine targets both the upper and lower body, combining gentle stretches for the shoulders and neck with movements that open the hips and stretch the legs. Ideal for improving flexibility and relieving tension, it's a balanced practice to support overall mobility and relaxation.

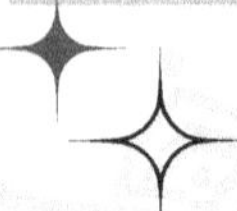

# Chapter 6: Eating for Energy and Weight Loss

## Healthy Eating Tips for Seniors

To maintain energy and support weight loss, seniors should focus on incorporating a variety of **nutrient-dense foods** into their diet. This means choosing foods that are rich in vitamins, minerals, and other nutrients important for health, while being relatively low in calories. **Fruits and vegetables** are excellent examples, providing essential vitamins and minerals, as well as fiber, which can help you feel full and satisfied. Aim for a colorful plate, as different colors represent different nutrients. For instance, dark leafy greens are high in calcium and iron, while berries are packed with antioxidants.

**Whole grains** are another key component of a healthy diet for seniors. Foods like quinoa, brown rice, and whole wheat bread are high in fiber, which aids in digestion and can help manage weight by keeping you fuller for longer periods. When choosing grains, always opt for whole grains over refined grains to ensure you're getting the full range of nutrients.

**Protein** is crucial for maintaining muscle mass, especially for seniors engaging in chair yoga or other forms of exercise. Lean sources of protein such as chicken, turkey, fish, beans, and legumes not only provide energy but also support muscle repair and growth. Including a source of lean protein in every meal can help balance blood sugar levels, which is important for weight management.

**Healthy fats** should not be overlooked. Avocados, nuts, seeds, and olive oil contribute healthy fats that are essential for brain health and can help absorb vitamins. However, it's important to consume these in moderation due to their high-calorie content.

**Hydration** plays a pivotal role in energy levels and weight loss. Seniors often experience a reduced sense of thirst, which can lead to dehydration. Drinking water throughout the day is crucial; aim for at least 8 glasses of water daily. Incorporating foods with high water content, such as cucumbers, tomatoes, and watermelon, can also contribute to hydration.

**Limiting processed foods and sugars** is beneficial for overall health and weight management. Processed foods often contain unhealthy fats, added sugars, and high levels of sodium, which can contribute to weight gain and other health issues. Instead, focus on whole, unprocessed foods for meals and snacks.

**Portion control** is another key aspect of eating for energy and weight loss. As metabolism slows with age, seniors might not need as many calories as they used to. Listening to your body's hunger cues and using smaller plates can help manage portion sizes without feeling deprived.

**Regular meal times** can help regulate your body's hunger signals and energy levels throughout the day. Skipping meals can lead to overeating later, so it's important to eat at consistent times. Additionally, incorporating healthy snacks between meals can prevent excessive hunger and help maintain steady blood sugar levels.

**Supplements** might be necessary for some seniors, especially if you're deficient in certain vitamins or minerals. However, it's best to get nutrients from food whenever possible. If you're considering supplements, consult with a healthcare provider to ensure they're appropriate for your needs.

By focusing on these dietary guidelines, seniors can support their energy levels and weight loss goals while enjoying a variety of delicious and nutritious foods. Remember, making small changes gradually is more sustainable than attempting a complete diet overhaul overnight. Start by incorporating one or two of these tips into your daily routine and build from there.

## Understanding Hydration's Importance

Hydration is a critical component of maintaining optimal health, especially for seniors who may not always recognize the signs of dehydration. As we age, our body's ability to conserve water decreases, and the sensation of thirst becomes less pronounced. This can lead to a reduced intake of fluids, making dehydration a common issue among the elderly population. It's important to understand that water plays a vital role in nearly every bodily function. It aids in digestion, helps transport nutrients and oxygen to cells, regulates body temperature, and acts as a lubricant for joints and tissues. For seniors engaging in chair yoga and other physical activities aimed at weight loss and improved fitness, staying adequately hydrated is essential to ensure that the body functions efficiently and to enhance the benefits of these activities.

**Dehydration** can have significant negative effects on the body, including increased risk of urinary tract infections, kidney stones, and even kidney failure. It can also lead to electrolyte imbalances, which can affect heart rhythm and muscle function. Furthermore, dehydration can exacerbate chronic conditions such as diabetes and heart disease. Recognizing the signs of dehydration is crucial. These can include dry mouth, fatigue, dizziness, less frequent urination, and dark-colored urine. If any of these symptoms are observed, it's important to increase fluid intake immediately.

For seniors practicing chair yoga, maintaining hydration can help improve flexibility, reduce the risk of muscle cramps and injuries, and promote better recovery after exercise. Water helps to keep the muscles and joints lubricated, making it easier to move and stretch. It also plays a role in regulating body temperature during physical activity, preventing overheating.

To ensure adequate hydration, seniors should aim to drink at least 8 glasses of water a day, or more if they are active or if the weather is hot. However, it's also important to listen to your body and drink when thirsty. Including foods with high water content in your diet, such as fruits and vegetables, can also help meet hydration needs. Watermelon, strawberries, cucumbers, and lettuce are excellent choices that can contribute to fluid intake.

In addition to water, other beverages like herbal teas and clear broths can contribute to daily fluid intake. However, it's advisable to limit the consumption of caffeinated beverages and alcohol, as these can lead to dehydration. For those who might find plain water unappealing, adding a slice of lemon, lime, or cucumber can enhance the flavor, making it more enjoyable to drink throughout the day.

It's also worth noting that certain medications and health conditions may affect hydration needs. Some medications can increase urination, while conditions such as diabetes can lead to increased fluid loss. Seniors with these considerations should discuss their hydration needs with a healthcare provider to ensure they're drinking enough to stay hydrated.

Incorporating hydration reminders into daily routines can be helpful. Setting reminders to drink water every hour or associating drinking water with specific activities, such as after completing a series of chair yoga poses, can ensure consistent fluid intake throughout the day. Keeping a water bottle within reach during the day can also encourage more frequent sips, gradually increasing overall water consumption.

Understanding the importance of hydration and implementing strategies to maintain adequate fluid intake are essential steps for seniors to support their overall health, enhance the effectiveness of physical activities like chair yoga, and promote successful weight loss efforts. By prioritizing hydration, seniors can improve their physical performance, protect against the negative effects of dehydration, and enjoy a higher quality of life.

# Download Your Gift

Scan the QR code and enjoy the gifts